enLIGHTened

enLIGHTened

How I Lost 40 Pounds with a Yoga Mat, Fresh Pineapples, and a Beagle-Pointer

by

Jessica Berger Gross

Illustrations by

Bobby Clennell

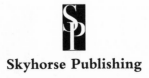

Skyhorse Publishing

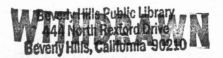

Skyhorse Publishing books may be purchased in bulk at special discounts
for sales promotion, corporate gifts, fund-raising, or educational purposes.
Special editions can also be created to specifications. For details, contact the
Special Sales Department, Skyhorse Publishing, 555 Eighth Avenue, Suite
903, New York, NY 10018 or info@skyhorsepublishing.com.

www.skyhorsepublishing.com

10 9 8 7 6 5 4 3 2 1

Library of Congress Cataloging-in-Publication Data

Gross, Jessica Berger.
  Enlightened : how I lost 40 pounds with a yoga mat, fresh pineapples,
and a beagle-pointer / Jessica Berger Gross.
    p. cm.
  ISBN 978-1-60239-639-5
  1. Weight loss. 2. Yoga. 3. Self-control. I. Title.
  RM222.2.G736 2009
  613.2'5--dc22
                                    2009000237

Printed in the United States of America

For Lucien

Contents

Preface

Twenty of us teenagers—converging from penthouse apartments on Park Avenue and public housing in the Bronx, from "broken" homes in Montclair, New Jersey, and small towns in West Virginia—sat together on the hardwood floor of a community hall in rural Pennsylvania. We'd come to attend a summer drama program for high school students.

Tara, the school's movement teacher, wore a long brown braid down her back. Movement class made me nervous. I was overweight and awkward in my body. One morning early on, Tara stood up at the front of the group of students and teachers and began demonstrating a series of exercises. Without music or counts, led only by her breath, she folded forward, bringing her head down to her knees, jumped back into a push-up, slid her chest up, climbed back into an inverted V-shape, and then stepped forward, first with her right leg and then her left, before landing back and folding forward once more.

This was 1987. I was from Long Island, and I had no idea what on earth Tara was doing. Was this some sort of religious cult I'd wandered into? Tara *looked* like she might be praying; there was something sacred-seeming about her movements. After watching Tara go through them once more, we tried them ourselves. She broke the components down one by one. Here, the forward bend. There, what she called a "downward dog."

Over the coming weeks, we learned to link our breath to the postures and to call them "sun salutations." With a big breath in we'd sweep our arms up overhead and exhale as we bent forward. Another inhalation to arch our backs and look up and then an exhalation to propel us back into a plank position and on from there. Soon, I was flying. It didn't matter how much I weighed.

For the first time in my life, at age fourteen, I felt whole. I wouldn't rediscover that feeling of wholeness for years, but when I did—more or less by accident—I recognized it immediately. This is what would save me, what would heal me.

This was yoga.

٭

The next time I encountered the sun salutations I was twenty and spending a college semester abroad in Nepal. I'd seen a flyer for a yoga center on the other side of Katmandu. One Saturday afternoon, a friend and I decided to go. The class, taught by a young man from India, was attended by middle-class and middle-aged Nepalese—teachers and accountants and stay-at-home moms looking to cure run-of-the-mill aches and pains.

We began with the sun salutations. Afterward, our teacher taught us some of the standing poses: tree pose, triangle pose, and then seated forward bends and twists like cobbler's pose and a simple seated twist. Ahh. There it was again. That *feeling*. That sense of belonging in my body—a sense of lightness. All those comforting tuna melts and plates of french fries; the parties and joints and beers; the misguided crushes and tentative sexual encounters—nothing could compare.

Fast-forward five more years. I was twenty-five and living in New York City. My boyfriend had dumped me, and my relationship with my family was as dysfunctional as ever. I was *this* close to becoming seriously can't-get-out-of-bed, about-to-gain-a-bunch-more-weight depressed. Somehow, instead of picking up a dinner of bagels and cream cheese and crawling onto my couch as I usually did when I was sad or stressed out, I used what willpower I could muster and dragged myself to a yoga center I'd been eyeing in my East Village neighborhood. Some part of me remembered those sun salutations and how they'd made me feel.

I was scared about going because I'd seen a lot of glamorous, thin types hanging out by the entryway doors. I hadn't worked out in over a year. Feeling self-conscious, I walked up the stairs, paid my attendance fee, and signed my name to the class roster. Cubbies were filled with coats and shoes—tall brown boots and Converse sneakers and other assorted downtown footwear. Farther in, the walls of the center were painted purple and turquoise and bright pink. In each of the practice rooms there was an altar decorated with framed photographs. An image of Gandhi, photos of Kennedy and Dr. Martin Luther King, Jr., another of the Dalai Lama—and pictures of a bunch of Indian men and women I didn't recognize. Were they saints? Teachers? Some advanced-looking students wearing Sanskrit-inscribed scarves and silver jewelry were drinking tea in a narrow hallway. I waited with the others who, like me, had come for the beginners' class. Our young, curly-haired teacher entered the room with a bunch of flowers, placed them at the altar, and lit a stick of incense, turning the lights down before taking her seat on the floor.

"OMMMM," the teacher chanted.

"Ommmm," the class responded in a low hum.

"Om," I whispered.

Again came the sun salutations I'd learned from Tara. Next were the standing poses, like warrior and tree pose, and the forward bends—all of which I'd encountered in Katmandu. My body remembered. Toward the end of class we paired up with classmates and worked on beginning backbends. My partner, a decidedly dewy woman I imagined to be an actress or dancer, and who didn't seem much like a "beginner" at all, encouraged me as I lay on my back, bent my knees, and held my ankles with my hands before lifting my chest up into a bridge pose.

The feeling of my breath and the opening up of my body was once again a revelation. (Yes, I'm a slow learner.) It wasn't simply that my body felt good in the stretches but that I felt like I was tapping into something special, something mystical.

"Is this really your first class?" my partner asked. "You're a natural."

I smiled back. I'd never felt like a natural at anything before.

All the bad stuff disappeared in that backbend—for the moment, at least. There was more to me than my depression, my struggles with weight, and my troubled relationships. I returned to class two days later. And again, two days after that. Every time I went, my *om* grew a little louder.

Eventually, my life changed, and my world—my heart—opened up. Yours can, too. This is the story of how studying yoga—not just the physical poses, but the philosophy behind them—helped me lose forty pounds, overcome my battle with depression, and change my life for good. In the coming chapters I'll share with you the basic principles of everyday living, eating, and moving that a decade of practicing yoga (and teaching it on and off) has taught me. Integrating these lessons into your life can lead you down the path of weight loss, help you find a sense of inner peace and contentment, and even—just maybe—a little bit of enlightenment.

A Note to the Reader

Some of my favorite yoga teachers begin class with brief discussions of yoga philosophy. The key text of yoga philosophy is called the Yoga Sutras, and it was written many years ago by a guru named Patañjali. The Sutras were originally written in the ancient language of Sanskrit, but they've been translated into English and other languages by contemporary yoga philosophers, who often add their own commentaries.

I begin each chapter of this book with a sutra in the original Sanskrit (minus the accents), so you can get a sense for what it looks and sounds like. Then I follow it up with a modern-day translation. Each translation puts its own spin on the teaching.

enLIGHTened

1

why i needed to get enlightened

SUTRA I.I: *ATHA YOGANUSANAM*

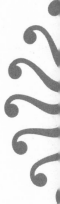

With prayers for divine blessings, now begins an exposition of the sacred art of yoga. —B. K. S. Iyengar

I n second grade, a boy in my class dubbed me "Bubble Berger." It was a terrible nickname, but in many ways it was fitting. I spent most of my childhood encased in a bubble of extra fat.

I grew up in the suburbs. My dad worked at a community college and my mom was an English teacher in our local public school. Life was hectic for my parents, and it took a toll on what we ate. All of us—including my two older brothers—struggled with weight. Two full-time jobs, plus ferrying three kids around from activity to activity, meant that mealtime was about filling up quickly on whatever was easiest for my mother to prepare. Some nights we'd have meat

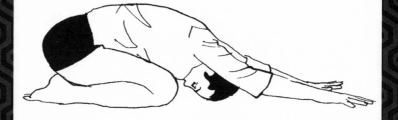

Sit on your heels, bring your feet together, and spread your knees apart. Lower your torso between your knees, and stretch your arms forward on the floor. Rest your forehead on the floor. (If it's difficult for you to be in this position comfortably, place your forehead on a folded blanket. You may also roll a blanket and place it between the back of your thighs and heels for extra support.)

and a starch: meatballs and spaghetti; hamburger patties or hot dogs on a bun; chicken or meatloaf or stuffed cabbage and baked potatoes or frozen fries. Other nights, when my mom was particularly tired or harried, dinner was what she called "catch as catch can"—usually a huge quantity of pasta with tomato sauce served straight out of the can. Sometimes we did takeout—pizza or Chinese food. Snacks filled up the kitchen pantry for the hungry afterschool hours. Our cupboards were stocked with pretzels, potato chips, and cookies; our freezer, with ice cream and frozen pizza.

I realized later that our diet wasn't all about convenience. Home wasn't a happy place. My father had a temper, and though much of the time he was a sweet and involved parent, buying me ballet shoes and driving me home from Hebrew school, on other days he turned mean. He hit me, and he hit my mother sometimes, too.

My mother, willing to do anything to keep her marriage intact, stayed. For her, as for me, eating was a form of comfort. Those simple carbohydrates acted like an anesthetic, and the fat we wore was a protective layer against the physical and emotional pain.

Hershey's Kisses, Pretzel Rods, and *Phil Donahue*

During the school year, my mother would come home from teaching completely drained. With the back screen door propped open, she'd carry groceries in from the car and, in a tired and slightly annoyed voice, ask me to take in the garbage cans from the street, walk the dog, help her put away the food. There was always something to do, and she was desperate for a break. She found it in junk food. Instead of consciously deciding on a snack and placing the food on a plate—where she'd be able to see exactly how much she was about to eat—she'd open a bag of pretzel rods and another of chocolate kisses, setting them beside her as she tucked herself into the couch for her favorite talk shows. Without taking her gaze off the television screen, she'd reach her hand into the bags for just a little something to tide her over before she had to start cooking dinner, a comforting treat to reward herself for a hard day at work. Before she knew it, she'd made a huge dent in each bag—and eaten many hundreds of calories. Stuffed, ashamed of having overindulged, and with her diet blown, she hardly felt like getting up to go make a healthy and satisfying dinner. And so, compounding the self-defeating cycle, she'd resign herself to putting up some water for a box of pasta and head back to the couch for more TV before starting her grading.

From a young age, I was a chubby kid. I avoided sports and playground activities and spent my recesses sitting on a tree stump reading novels. (The ballet shoes my father bought me didn't get much use.) I never made the connection between what was going on at home, my eating habits, and my expanding waistline. Since my parents were overweight, and both of my brothers were a bit on the husky side, I figured it was my unhappy genetic destiny to carry around extra pounds.

Then one day in eighth grade, I came across *The Sweet Dreams Body Book: A Guide to Diet, Nutrition, and Exercise* by Julie Davis. Davis advocated portion control, exercise, and increasing your intake of fruits and vegetables. I'm not sure how the book landed in my hands. Maybe my mother bought it for me? I do remember staying up all night glued to its every word. There seemed to be a way out of my bubbly misery!

Over the next few months, the book became my bible. I ate carrot sticks and rice cakes and watched my portions. And I lost a lot of weight—about twenty pounds. My mother, delighted and proud of the new pretty me, took me shopping for new clothes. Adorned in my fitted black stirrup pants, I came out of my shell at school and made more friends.

Although I loved, loved, loved being thin, I didn't manage to stay that way for long. My *Sweet Dreams* diet was just that—a diet, a temporary fix. I didn't know how to maintain the change long-term. Underneath the new clothes and slim body, I was still the same old unhappy me with the same set of problems.

～

My mother went on periodic diets, too. Her weight would creep up higher and higher until she had to shop in the special section of her favorite department store where they kept the plus sizes. Eventually, she'd sign up for Weight Watchers, attending weekly meetings and weigh-ins, and she'd make the switch from pasta to turkey burgers—hold the bun—and chicken with steamed broccoli—sauce on the side—from the local Chinese takeout. After a couple of months of dedication and deprivation, the pounds would fall away. My mother's spirit seemed lighter when she lost weight, and she looked younger, too. She colored her graying hair a light brown and bought a stylish new wardrobe from the "regular" women's section—lots of Liz Claiborne—in sizes 10 and 12 and 14.

But then the once-weekly special treat—a chocolate frozen yogurt dessert (low in calories but high in sugars and carbohydrates)—would become a daily, and then twice-daily, fixture, and pasta would wind its way back into the dinner rotation. It didn't take long for my mom to return to her old ways. She'd slide back up the scale and out of the clothes she'd splurged on.

Unconsciously, I mimicked her behavior. When I was between diets in elementary and middle school, my guilty pleasure was chocolate ice cream or potato chips or pistachio nuts—fattening, comforting foods I'd pour into bowls downstairs in the kitchen and then run up to my room to eat in private. Since the snacks were in my family's pantry, it didn't seem like they could be *that* bad for me.

As a teenager I yo-yoed between normal and chubby and just plain fat. I made friends with the older, thin, stylish drama club girls in high school, emulating them in all sorts of ways but never learning to copy their eating habits. After school, I'd come home and snack on bagels and cream cheese. Occasionally, I'd have an apple or some grapes, but the idea of basing my diet on fruits and vegetables and whole grains couldn't have been further from my mind. I was just trying to survive high school, and my family. *The Sweet Dreams Body Book* was aimed at preteens, and I jammed it toward the back of my bookshelf. At night I'd sit in my bedroom, stuffing myself with chips, smoking cigarettes out the window, reading novels, studying, and memorizing my guidebook to college admissions, which seemed to be the only ticket out of my parents' house.

Meanwhile, there were plenty of opportunities for overeating. I worked as a cashier at a Japanese restaurant. During my shift, I'd grab handfuls of rice cracker mix from the bar when nobody was looking. When we closed for the night I'd go to town on the free meal offered to the staff. Who could pass up free teriyaki and tempura? (Never mind that it was my second dinner of the day.) Similarly, when my friends and I weren't caging wine coolers and cans of Bud from the local Dairy Barn drive-through window, we'd spend nights out at the Golden Reef Diner—a classic greasy spoon coffee shop, New York style—where I ate mozzarella sticks or cheese fries between cigarettes. I poured whole milk and gobs of sugar into bottomless cups of coffee. Once we could drive, a friend and I made a ritual of weekly dinners at Pizzeria Uno, meals that began with a large platter of cheese nachos and went on from there.

By twelfth grade, the clothes in my closet no longer fit. I had trouble coming up with workable outfits in the morning and went on an embarrassed solo mission to the mall to buy oversized baggy jeans from the men's section of the Gap. I hid in them and in long flowing skirts and big black mock-turtle-neck tops.

Around this time my mother started having health troubles. No one said it aloud, but my brothers and I knew that the problem was her weight. One morning she was rushed to the hospital complaining of heart palpitations and chest pain and was diagnosed with high blood pressure, a heart condition, and type 2 diabetes. That summer I ate my way through the pain and grief and fear of losing her. I left for college at the end of the summer, thirty pounds overweight.

～

At Vassar, I made friends with the cool New York City private school girls. I wasn't sure why they included me in their group—I always felt like the frumpy fat friend. (And then there was my financial aid package and work-study job, which further set me apart.) Despite my friends' example, I didn't do anything to change my diet, and my weight continued to yo-yo. But I figured that the pizza I ate several nights a week couldn't be much of a problem since my skinny roommate was eating it, too. Never mind that I ate twice as much as she did. When she'd have a slice or two, I'd have three. Okay, maybe four.

At lunch I ordered french fries to go with my sandwich, and no weekend morning was complete without bagels and eggs, college-cafeteria style. Even when I ate Sunday brunch with my one super-healthy and together friend, Jenna, a dancer, I'd pile onto my tray mounds of cream cheese, a toasted bagel or two, and a plate with a cheese omelet and hash browns. I took a women's studies class, became convinced that fat was a feminist issue, and vowed never to subscribe to any patriarchal beauty myth. I protested sexism one french fry at a time.

Of course, I *did* care. My weight went up and down the scale, depending on my mood and pizza consumption, who I was or wasn't dating, and how bad things were going with my family back home—but I was always fifteen to forty pounds heavier than I should have been. When I was a sophomore in college, my eldest brother got married. I was a bridesmaid in his fancy wedding at the Rainbow Room in New York wearing a size-16 dress that had to be special-ordered.

Everything changed for me when I signed up for spring semester abroad during my junior year. I wanted adventure, to go to a developing country in Africa or Asia. My mother wanted me to be safe. We compromised on what was, at the time, the peaceful nation of Nepal, sandwiched between India and China.

I packed my black-on-black wardrobe and my poetry journals. Although I did some reading on Nepali culture, I really had no idea what to expect. When I got to the airport to meet up with my fellow students in the program, it dawned on me that there might be a reason why they all had hiking boots and polar fleece paraphernalia. The mountains in Nepal were serious business, and most of my classmates had chosen Nepal because they wanted to trek through the Himalayas.

The idea of the program was that we students were to travel around the country by bus and by foot, getting to know Nepal, its language, culture, and people. After a short time in the Katmandu Valley, we began the trek to the village where we'd all be doing homestays. Like many places in the Nepali countryside, it was only accessible by footpath. We took a bus until the road ended, and then started walking. I seriously thought I might die—not because trekking in Nepal was dangerous but because I'd never walked that much in my life. We spent day after day hiking, bunking at teahouses along the way. Lucky for me, the other students took me under their wings, and rather than resent me for slowing the group down, they cheered me on. Stopping for breaks only prolonged the trip, so I put one foot in front of the next and slowly made my way up and down those mountains.

That first trek was just the beginning. In Nepal, walking was a fact of life. My Katmandu homestay family lived next to the Monkey Temple, more than an hour's walk from the schoolhouse where I took daily classes. Later, I trekked for five full days and back, just me and a local guide, to a Buddhist nunnery. Not only did I get thin, even better, I got strong and healthy.

Meanwhile, my diet couldn't have been healthier if a personal chef from the Canyon Ranch health spa had accompanied me abroad. The typical Nepali meal of *dahl baht*—eaten for lunch and dinner—consists of generous heaps of simply prepared vegetables and rice and lentils, sometimes with a thin whole wheat bread, or *chapatti*, thrown in for good measure.

My program mates also cajoled me into cutting down my smoking dramatically—from a pack to a cigarette or two a day. My efforts here were helped along by Nepali custom, as it wasn't acceptable for a young woman to be seen smoking in public. (Who knew patriarchy could sometimes work in your favor?) We didn't do much drinking, either.

Here's a recipe for a mild but flavorful *dahl*—or lentil dish—to make at home that comes from Chindi Varadarajulu, the owner of my favorite neighborhood Indian restaurant, Chutney Villa, in Vancouver, British Columbia. You'll need to shop at an Indian grocery store for some of the ingredients.

Dahl with Spinach

1 cup of mung beans (*moong dahl*), rinsed thoroughly

1 bunch of spinach

6 cloves of garlic, crushed with skin on

1 teaspoon black mustard seed

1 teaspoon fennel seeds

2 sprigs of curry leaves

1 medium onion (thinly sliced)

2 tablespoons coconut oil or vegetable oil

2 sprigs of cilantro

After rinsing the beans, put them in a pot with 3 or 4 cups of water. Add the garlic. Bring to a rolling boil for about 5 minutes and then turn down the heat and let simmer till the *dahl* is cooked soft. This will take about 20 minutes. By now most of the water should be gone and the *dahl* should have a very thick, porridge-like consistency.

Chop your spinach and add it to the *dahl*; add salt to taste. Simmer for 5 minutes more and remove from stove.

In a pan heat the oil. When hot add the mustard and fennel seeds. When the seeds start to pop, add the onion and curry leaves. Cook till the onions turn a nice golden brown. Remove from the stove and pour this over the *dahl* mixture and give it a stir. Garnish with cilantro and serve with rice (or *roti* for the advanced—a thin, whole wheat, tortilla-like Indian bread).

I fell in love with the feeling that came from moving my body, with the high of eating a healthy meal after a long, physically-active, emotionally-satisfying day. I hiked through the countryside with my classmates and teachers and attended that yoga class in Katmandu. Back in the schoolhouse, my friend and I practiced the movements we'd learned in class.

Between the trekking, the daily walks, my new vegetarian diet, and the yoga, I couldn't help but lose weight. Soon my culturally appropriate long skirts fell off my hips, and I drowned in my formerly fitted T-shirts. I emerged from that semester certifiably, unequivocally, and for the first time since I was twelve—thin.

Something else happened, too. Trekking one day on my own, after a hard morning's climb, the sun shining, the green hills dotted with grazing animals, my body more vital and alive than ever before, something touched me. It was something deep within me yet simultaneously beaming down from that blue sky. This might sound crazy to some, but I felt at one with God. I felt wrapped up in love and had the sense that, although my family life might be troubled, I would somehow, eventually, find a way out.

～

Back at Vassar my senior year, the reaction to the new, thin me was more overwhelming than I could have imagined. My friends and acquaintances were shocked at the change. I'd lost close to thirty pounds and people, particularly straight men, treated me differently. Guys who hadn't been interested in me for three years were suddenly having a second look. I tried to take it all in and worked to keep up my healthy, active habits. During my senior year, and for a year or so after graduation, while traveling and working abroad, I hiked and walked and ate moderately and consciously. I managed to keep the weight off.

Then, I moved to New York. It wasn't as easy to stay healthy in the city. The ups and downs of the life of a twenty-something, the smoking and drinking with my friends (which I'd taken up again after leaving Nepal), a not-so-good-for-me boyfriend, a bout of unemployment, the complicated and dysfunctional relationship with my parents, and the fact that it seemed cheaper and easier to grab a bagel or make a bowl of pasta for dinner than to prepare a vegetable stir-fry in my minuscule kitchen all contributed to my gaining back the weight I'd lost.

After a couple of years of serious floundering when it came to my health, career, and relationships, I found myself at that yoga center one winter day. In that first class there was so much sweet silence. (Plus, I kept seeing celebrities like Christy Turlington, Russell Simmons, and Woody Harrelson in class, which didn't hurt either.) I kept going back for more. I quit smoking and became fanatical about going to class three times a week.

Soon after, I moved to Madison, Wisconsin, to attend graduate school. In Madison I continued practicing yoga and even began teaching small, informal classes—first to my friends at my hippie housing cooperative and then at a women's health club near campus. I made new friends who didn't obsess about the size of their clothes (they found most of them secondhand at thrift stores anyway) but were interested in eating good, local, mostly vegetarian food. During this time I was at a healthy weight—about a size eight—thanks to yoga, biking around town, and eating vegetarian. But I also smoked pot before bed almost every night to relax and got drunk most weekends. Although I had acquired some aspects of a healthy lifestyle, I didn't have my emotional life in order. I didn't yet understand that yoga wasn't just about doing the *asana* (the physical poses); it was also about following a broader set of principles and practices that would help me live consciously, with self-awareness.

During my second year in Madison I fell in love, for good, with Neil, a man as kind and as thoughtful as he was brilliant. We met in a sociology seminar where I initially developed a crush on our unavailable, much older professor. Despite the distraction of the crush, I managed to see that Neil was cute, and I was impressed by his comments in class—though I didn't always catch some of his more obscure intellectual references. But Neil had mentioned something about a girlfriend, and anyway, I really did like that professor.

When nothing, thankfully, came of that (not that I didn't try), Neil e-mailed me after winter break (by then he was single) and asked if I'd like to meet him for a coffee. He phoned that night, and we talked for more than an hour. His voice was kind, he got most of *my* references—except the pop culture ones—and he was a good listener, too.

"What did you do between 1996 and 1998?" he—seriously—wanted to know. Generally, the guys I'd dated couldn't have cared less about what I'd done that morning much less two years before.

We skipped the coffee and went sledding on our first date, taking turns sliding down a hill on a makeshift sled—a plastic piece from a dish rack Neil had rigged up. On the way home, it didn't matter that the heat in his car was broken or that my jeans were drenched from the snow. On our second date Neil took me to a free classical music concert at the university and then to a gay dance club in town that was having an eighties music night. We shared our first kiss in the middle of the dance floor. That weekend I invited him over to hang out with me at my co-op, and we stayed up all night, talking and kissing, going out for breakfast the next morning.

We'd marry two years later. Neil, I would later discover, is the rare kind of man who cooks, shares in child care, and manages to hold down a successful career, too. (His secret? Very little sleep and infrequent trips to the dentist.) Not that Neil's perfect; he needs to be convinced to do the bare minimum of self-care like a toenail trim or buying a new pair of jeans when his are literally in shreds. But he's funny and generous and—skip this if you're one of his academic colleagues—the best possible person to watch reality television with. He's an A+ husband.

Even though I'd lucked out in meeting Neil, I soon discovered that a good relationship is not a cure for unresolved emotional issues. Several months after we started dating, I crashed. Sometimes, things just have to get worse before they can get better. I was about to hit rock bottom, and my highest weight yet.

2

the rinse cycle

SUTRA I.33: *MAITRI KARUNA MUDITA UPEKSANAM*
SUKHA DUHKA PUNYA APUNYA VISAYANAM
BHAVANATAH CITTAPRASADANAM

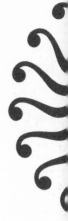

Undisturbed calmness of mind is attained by cultivating friendliness toward the happy, compassion for the unhappy, delight in the virtuous, and indifference toward the wicked.

—Swami Prabhavananda and Christopher Isherwood

Why I Stopped Speaking to My Parents

From a thousand miles away in Madison my relationship with my parents seemed better, but, really, we were as dysfunctional as ever. Phone calls were difficult to get through. During the worst of them, I'd hold the receiver a few inches from my ear and cry.

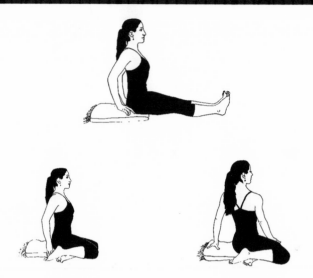

Sit on two folded blankets with your feet stretched out in front of you on the floor. Bend your legs and fold them to the right. Place your right ankle on top of the sole of the upturned left foot, so your right shin and left foot form a cross. Place your right hand on your left knee and place your left hand directly behind you on the floor or on a block. Sit up tall. Inhaling, lengthen up through your spine, and exhaling, twist toward the left—rotating your waist and chest. Turn your head and look behind you. Relax the muscles in your face and continue breathing deeply. To change sides, untwist and face center. Stretch your legs out in front of you again. Now bend your legs to the left and place your left hand on your right knee and repeat the pose, this time twisting to the right. Twists give you the chance to release and let go of what you no longer need to store inside.

After graduation, missing the city and perhaps subconsciously hoping to mend my relationship with my parents, I applied for jobs in New York. Neil stayed in Madison when I flew back for a week of job interviews, stopping first in Long Island for a weekend visit home.

My mother couldn't wait to show me her newly-renovated kitchen, her stainless steel appliances, her granite countertops. On Sunday morning, I opened the refrigerator and didn't hold onto the door. It swung wide open and banged against the cabinets, scratching the maple. My father was pissed but tried to keep his temper under control.

My mother was in the next room, anxiously working her way through a bag of pretzel rods and trying to look busy with the Sunday newspaper. I sat down at the computer. I needed to print my résumé and asked my father for help with the printer. He came over and told me to get up and give him the desk chair. After a minute, I went and sat down on the couch.

"Stay here," my father demanded, gritting his teeth. "I'm not going to slave away while you relax on the couch."

I wasn't used to being talked to like that anymore. "Don't tell me what to do," I said. "I'm an adult."

"You're an ungrateful bitch is what you are," he answered.

This time I wouldn't have it. I didn't need him. I had Neil. I had a graduate degree and five job interviews that week.

"Don't do this," I said. "I won't let you do this to me anymore."

"Do what? What have I ever done to you?" he said.

"You hit me," I screamed. The words rushed out before I could consider them. "And you hit her, too," I said, pointing to my mother.

She looked up at me, shocked that the words had been spoken. In my family, hitting a child could be rationalized as punishment, but hitting your wife was sick, something other people did.

"How many times?" my father yelled, looking at her. "How many times did I hit you?"

"Too many to count," I said. My mother nodded.

"And you hit me," I said. "I was just a kid."

"You were a selfish brat," he said.

"The first time you hit her," my mother said, "she was two and a half. She was still in diapers." I loved my mother for saying so but hated her more for staying married to him.

"Why didn't you leave?" I asked.

"Maybe I should have," she said.

"I made some mistakes," my father said. He was crying. "And I'm sorry I hurt you. But you were a difficult child." His eyes turned steely. "I've worked too hard to spend the rest of my life apologizing for what happened years ago."

We went back and forth for hours. Eventually, there was nothing left to say. I had to get out. My parents insisted on driving me to the city, where I'd stay with a friend. I was exhausted from crying and fighting and agreed to the ride. I sat in the backseat and wore headphones like an angry, helpless teenager.

My father and I got out of the car. "I love you," I said, giving my father a hug. "But don't call me. I'll let you know when I'm ready to talk."

I never was. I realized that my relationship with my parents was no good for me, no better than a relationship with an abusive husband. So why not end it? What outdated rule of familial obligation required me to continue having a relationship with them?

The break wasn't easy. A job offer materialized from all those interviews and Neil and I found an apartment in Brooklyn and moved in together. On paper, the position—a research job at NYU—sounded challenging and fulfilling, but the reality was that I spent my days alone in a tiny windowless room without colleagues or coworkers. The professors I worked for had offices elsewhere on campus. A week could go by without anyone knowing whether or not I even showed up. That probably would have been fine if I wasn't desperately sad and conflicted and guilt-ridden about my decision to stop speaking to my parents.

That fall and winter I ate and ate. I trudged from our Brooklyn apartment to the subway, picking up a bagel and coffee on the way. I wasn't pounding back bags of potato chips or ice cream sundaes—I tried eating at least *semi*-healthy foods. A bagel seemed harmless enough; I figured bread and cheese were wholesome ingredients. And what New Yorker *didn't* eat bagels? At night, I'd order up an entrée of tofu and broccoli from the vegetarian Chinese restaurant down the street, not seeing anything wrong with eating the entire oily dish in one sitting.

When we cooked, Neil would dish me up bowl after bowl of pasta just like my mother had done for me. At the office, I'd buy split pea or black bean soup from the gourmet delicatessen but unthinkingly accept the free roll that came with it. I'd also pick up a fruit smoothie, and though it said on the container that it was two servings, I'd down the whole thing with my lunch. To make matters worse, at night before bed—*every* night before bed—Neil and I had something we called a "snack" in the private language all couples have. For us, this was a seemingly innocuous mixture of Cheerios and chocolate chips. Sure, the portions were pretty small (although they grew bigger the more depressed I became), and, yes, the chips were organic, but the fact is that my bedtime ritual was distressingly similar to my mother's afternoon dips into a bag of Hershey's kisses. Combined with my big portions at dinner and my morning bagel with cream cheese, it was more than enough to make me gain weight despite attending yoga class regularly.

My standard work uniform that year was composed of forgiving sweaters and pants I bought at the Gap. I'd started out with size-8 trousers, and by January, I was wearing a size 12. When I dared to step on a scale I covered my eyes and peeked through my fingers, humiliated to see the number creeping toward 150. I'd gained twenty-five pounds in five months. At five feet two, it was as much as I'd weigh later when nine months pregnant.

I wasn't just overweight, though; I was clinically depressed. The break with my parents had brought back all of my childhood traumas. Life seemed pointless, not worth the effort. By winter, I couldn't get out of bed. I remember one last shot at normalcy—a New Year's Eve party thrown by an old friend. Neil convinced me that we should go, and I put on my least unflattering outfit (a black sweater and a skirt with an elastic waistband) and we took the subway in. I was ashamed to see my friend, to show her my body underneath my winter coat. I couldn't even stay until midnight. During the time, I developed some odd theories about weight.

Odd Theories About Weight

1. Wool trousers shrink over time (which explained why mine were too tight and needed replacing);

2. Attending yoga class three times a week meant I could eat whatever I wanted—and if I was *still* overweight after all that yoga, it was just my fate; and

3. Yoga is a cardio workout, so doing yoga gave me a free pass from the gym or hiking trail. (Later I'd learn that yoga paired with cardiovascular exercise is a truly ideal combination.)

That January things went further downhill. My depression turned from sadness and melancholy to dark desperation. It didn't matter that I wasn't in touch with my parents; my father returned each night in my nightmares. I'd wake up screaming, sweating. I escaped into fantasies about suicide and daydreamed about my funeral. And then I'd remember Neil, whose father had died the previous spring. I couldn't do that to him.

Since suicide was out of the question, my depressive thoughts turned to the idea of checking myself into a psychiatric hospital. I noted the small box advertisements in the *New Yorker* for McLean Hospital, where Susanna Kaysen and Sylvia Plath had been hospitalized. I imagined white cotton sheets, no responsibilities other than therapy sessions, small blue pills to pacify me, and endless, lazy afternoons spent chain-smoking in the patient lounge while the television played in the background.

After six months, I quit my job. Somehow I kept going to yoga, only missing class on my worst days. I'm not sure how I dragged myself there, but when I was able to get out of bed and into my yoga clothes and onto the subway from Brooklyn to Manhattan, my mood brightened—at least for that hour and a half of class.

I'd place my mat in my favorite spot in the practice room as the teacher turned on the pre-class music (anything from Indian chants to Peter Gabriel to The Beatles). We'd begin class in meditation with *oms* and chanting, and before long we'd start to move. Soon I'd be swept up in the wave of the sun salutations and lifted out of my otherwise all-consuming thoughts.

Was there a way to bring that feeling into my life the rest of the time as well? It dawned on me that there was; I would simply do more yoga. And who practices yoga all the time? Yoga teachers do! So I stopped daydreaming about suicide and started daydreaming about becoming a yoga teacher. My logic might have been faulty (as I'd later learn, it's not just the yoga asana but living according to the principles of yoga philosophy that generates a sustained sense of inner peace), but it was a step in the right direction. Still, I had my doubts.

Reasons Not to Become a Yoga Teacher

1. Teaching yoga doesn't exactly pay the bills (when I'd later teach at Canyon Ranch, I'd get paid $15 for an hour-long class; teachers who own their own centers or organize their own classes can make a more decent living);

2. I could barely make it out of bed, much less into a forearm stand; and

3. All the yoga teachers I knew were thin and at one with the universe. I wasn't either.

Nevertheless, one day, after a second bowl of pasta and a long cuddle on the couch, I brought the idea up with Neil. "I was thinking . . ." I said, under my breath.

"Hmmm?" Neil was checking his e-mail before bed, hoping to receive news of a job interview at one of the many universities to which he'd applied.

"I had an idea," I said, louder this time. "About what to do with my life."

"Great," Neil said. "Tell me." He was probably thinking law school—or maybe another nonprofit or research job. Perhaps I'd decided to apply to teach in the public schools?

"I was thinking that I'd like to be a yoga teacher."

Plunk. That was the sound of our combined household income plummeting.

"Fantastic, sweetie," said Neil. "That's an excellent idea!" He headed back to the dining room to work all night on his latest academic paper in the hopes that one of us might eventually be gainfully employed.

I Feel Pretty, Oh So Pretty

And so, overweight and depressed, I did what no unemployed person without a hefty trust fund should do. I signed up for a yoga teacher-training retreat in Mexico. The teacher was a smiling, muscular man named Baron Baptiste. Baron was raised by a couple of old-school yoga teachers in Southern California. As a young man he studied with yoga masters in the U.S. and India. After teaching in LA, he eventually opened up a popular yoga center in Cambridge, Massachusetts. Baron topped off his yoga-teacher-next-door shorts and T-shirt look with a rotating wardrobe of bandanas wrapped around his head. His style of yoga was athletic and unorthodox, his sweat-producing classes stoked by a heated room, feel-good music from Moby to Madonna, and a steady stream of New Age aphorisms. It may not have been straight-up classical yoga, but Baron and his style of yoga spoke to me. Sometimes, when you're feeling down, a good issue of *Us Weekly* can be more satisfying than a *New Yorker*. Baron would throw a wheatgrass-induced adage out there, leaving us to think it over while enduring our fifth full backbend. What he said had a way of sinking in.

One saying he returned to again and again was that we were lumps of clay, and what we needed was to find the beautiful sculpture inside the lump, like Michelangelo carving out his *David*. We needed, in other words, to discover our true and best selves. As we did this, though, we should keep our eyes on our own mat and not worry about anyone else's downward dog or arm balance or how deeply others in class seemed to be going in their meditation. Baron, who never minded a mixed metaphor, said we were children of God waiting to break out of our cocoons.

Late one afternoon toward the end of the retreat, Baron gathered us students together at the front of the yoga room after a long asana session. I'd already sweated my way through two changes of clothes that day, and I'd jotted down several life-changing, *utterly* profound quotes in the thick black journals Baron had handed us at the start of the training—scribbles that weeks later, when I referred back to them, made me wonder just what had been in that incense. But Baron's message resonated, and continues to resonate, with me. That afternoon, wanting us to explore more important things than our poses, he asked us to talk about how we saw ourselves and our bodies.

Opened up—not just physically, but emotionally, too—from a week of all-day yoga and evenings of meditation and contemplation, the students revealed themselves, sharing stories of eating disorders, starvation diets, and flirtations with bulimia. People also talked about the competitive vibe that can occasionally come up in yoga centers, where yoga poses are practiced in body-hugging leggings and revealing tank tops. Yogis are human, too, and in some classes, there's pressure to be thin, even to have the right outfit on. I had a different realization. As unsure of myself as I felt in the rest of the world, the yoga room was the one place where I felt beautiful, where I'd forget all my self-doubt and the extra weight I carried. Once I realized this, I just had to testify.

I stood up in the front of the room. My voice was shaky, but my speech was determined and heartfelt. "Growing up, I was always the friend, the sidekick, the one who wore baggy black sweaters and Doc Martens, who had crushes on my friends' boyfriends, the one who'd end up crying on street corners, drunk and lonely on the Lower East Side at 2 A.M. But when I practice yoga, I feel beautiful."

I know, I know. Doc Martens, Lower East Side, 2 A.M.? A yoga retreat in Mexico? Please, cue the harmoniums and light some Nag Champa incense. But here's the thing: The sentiment was real. I had been down-on-my-knees depressed, and in the yoga room, I *did* feel beautiful. Still, it was embarrassing to say aloud. Me, beautiful? Overweight, out of shape, depressed me? But the other yogis went wild, offering me hugs, applause, after-dinner foot rubs.

While it was heartening to know that the yoga community would accept me at a larger weight, I knew I wanted to change.

For one thing, there were many poses I just couldn't do because of my size. Getting up into a handstand—no matter how many times Baron helped me kick up—proved impossible; I weighed too much to balance my entire body weight on my arms. Ditto for balancing in headstand. This is not to say that a bigger person can't practice these poses—some do, beautifully—but for *me*, and for my body, the weight really did get in the way. When I'd attempt a deep, detoxifying twist, the extra flesh around my midsection would keep me from going as far as I otherwise might.

Baron knew that, when it came to our physical and emotional well-being, what we ate mattered—and that a healthy diet was as important as regular yoga practice. In

Mexico, he served us the sort of high-fiber foods I wasn't used to cooking, much less digesting: an assortment of lentils and beans, local fruits, avocados and greens and quinoa and whole grains, nothing industrially processed or packaged. In addition to the fiber, Baron encouraged us to eat sparingly; for a couple days in the middle of the week he even limited the amount of grains and lentils offered and upped the quantity of fruits and vegetables we were served. My system went into hard-core detoxification mode. I was pooping my brains out, and I felt fantastic. I even—temporarily—lost weight.

The yoga retreat in Mexico was Neil's gift to me, a last-ditch attempt to pull me out of my depression and out of our Brooklyn bed. But when it was over it was back to real life. In Mexico, I realized that—no surprise—my unresolved feelings about my parents were at the core of my depression. I knew, too, that Neil and I couldn't go on living in an expensive city like New York when neither of us had a full-time job there. (Again, not rocket science!) Neil and I talked—pillow talk, really—about heading to the woods for a year, to live as cheaply as we could while we figured out our next steps, both emotionally and career-wise.

As the yoga gods would have it, while I was in Mexico Neil got the call offering him a one-year visiting professor job at a liberal arts college in the Berkshire Mountains of Massachusetts. While changing locations isn't a solution to your problems—they call it "pulling a geographic" in AA—I couldn't help but see the chance to move as a sign. What better place to work on getting healthy than in the country? Fresh air, nature, and a salary with health insurance. Plus, I liked the idea of getting my yoga teaching career off the ground in a place that might not be overflowing with other yoga teachers. On a visit to the area after I returned from Mexico, we found a small, charming house to rent in a rural town twenty-five minutes away from the college.

That's how it came to be that I traded in my former professional wardrobe of uncomfortably tight trousers and sensible flats for an old pair of snow boots, a new pair of Birkenstock sandals, and an oversized parka. I let my MetroCard expire and hoped to teach yoga while I figured out what to do with my life.

New England was peaceful and pretty, but a few days after the moving van headed back to Brooklyn, I realized that the nearest yoga class for me to take was many miles away from our house. There I was—no more Baron, no more yoga center with inspiring teachers handing out chant sheets and rubbing my temples with oil at the end of class. I'd have to be my own teacher. If I wanted that yoga high, I'd have to conjure it up on my own. With no other choice, I rolled out my yoga mat, dusted off my yoga asana and philosophy books, and started up a personal home practice in my pajamas.

3

truthfulness (*satya*)

WAKE UP AND SMELL THE GREEN TEA
(SATYA: TRUTH, SINCERITY, GENUINENESS,
HONESTY, VIRTUOUSNESS)

SUTRA II.36: *SATYAPRATISTHAYAM*
KRIYAPHALASRAYATVAM

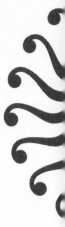

A student of yoga ought
to be a follower of truth in thought,
speech, and action. —Geeta Iyengar

Keeping It Real

Sometime between 500 and 200 BC, the Indian scholar and all-around holy man Patañjali compiled a series of philosophical tenets previously passed down orally from teacher to student. Each tenet, or *sutra*, is concise—only a few words or sentences—yet packed with insight, like a Frank Rich column. These tenets have become known as the Yoga Sutras, and today, serious yogis take them as their guide to asana practice and to life. At several points in the text, Patañjali discusses the notion of *satya*, or truthfulness, and says that countless benefits come to those who practice it.

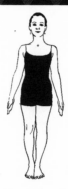

This chapter is about becoming more truthful in everything you do, including what you're eating and why. Mountain pose is the perfect posture to practice as you explore this Yoga Sutra. Stand with your arms extended down at your sides, your chest open, and your chin held parallel to the ground. Notice the feeling of your feet on the floor; spread them wide, stretching through the toes and heels. Separate and spread your toes. From there, let your attention gradually move up your body. Engage your thigh muscles and allow your tailbone to tuck slightly. Drop the tops of your shoulders down your back and spread your chest wide. Let your head balance on top of your neck as if held in place by puppet strings descending from the ceiling. Now add the sweep of your breath into the posture—breathing up from the floorboards through your feet and legs, into your spine, through your chest, and exhaling one long smooth breath. Hold for several cycles of breath, feeling taller and more expanded with each inhalation and exhalation. Standing in this pose, imagine yourself becoming more open and expanded—and genuine and truthful—on the inside too.

In his translation of the Sutras, yoga luminary B. K. S. Iyengar defines truthfulness as sincerity, genuineness, honesty, and virtuousness. "When the seeker is firmly established in the practice of truth," he translates Patañjali as saying, "his words become so potent that whatever he says comes to realization." Of course, lots of spiritual traditions emphasize the need to be truthful; think of the Ten Commandments and "Thou shall not bear false witness." But Patañjali's understanding of the concept is different. For him, truthfulness isn't just about what we say, but how genuinely and authentically we live every aspect of our lives. And let's face it: When it comes to eating and exercise, many of us are anything but "firmly established in the practice of truth." We fool ourselves about what we put into our mouths, why we eat the way we do, and how much exercise we get. For me, the first step on the road to getting thin was waking up to the truth about my eating and exercise habits.

"Why Do You Eat So Much?"

It all started with a little humiliation. It was summer in the Berkshires; Neil was to begin his teaching job that September. Our rented white clapboard house had a side porch and three upstairs bedrooms and inspiring bucolic views. We set up a bare-bones household: a table and chairs, a couch, a bed. We woke to the sound of roosters.

The more we lead a life of honesty, the more we will see the results.

—Sri Swami Satchidananda

Every morning that summer, I got on my yoga mat. I was unsure of myself; I'd hardly ever practiced yoga on my own, without a teacher or friend to encourage me. For inspiration, I listened to Indian chants sung by Krishna Das, a musician from the Long Island suburbs, like me, who had found his guru in India decades before, in the 1960s. "Hare Krishna," he'd sing, and I'd hum along.

On the other side of the room, by a window that looked out onto our lawn and small pond, I set up my computer on a plain wooden table and began writing for yoga magazines. I rented space for next to nothing in the basement of a community center in the nearby college town and made flyers advertising a yoga class. The college where Neil worked hired me to teach a class to their faculty and staff, and another to students.

Sounds good, right? Like I was on the right track?

Well, although I *was* headed in the right direction, the scale didn't register it yet. The truth was, I was heavier than ever. While I'd made drastic changes to my work and living situations—quit my job, moved to the country—I couldn't get out of the bad eating habits I'd reverted to the year before. I wasn't snacking on crazy amounts of junk food, but I was eating way too much, and the wrong things.

And then summer houseguests started arriving, and I couldn't avoid the truth anymore. Rex (some names changed to protect the innocent), a friend from graduate school who'd grown up in rural Minnesota, was the first. He drove up in a rented convertible for an unexpectedly rainy weekend with his new girlfriend Christina, a petite twenty-something from Queens whom he'd met on the subway during morning rush hour. Although not exactly impolite, Christina was one of those people who couldn't help but say whatever popped into her head. During Sunday brunch at one of our new favorite restaurants, Christina ordered pancakes off the children's menu, while I wolfed down an entire three-egg omelet with hash browns and toast. It *sounded* healthier, somehow, than pancakes or waffles. But while she had a couple of bites before putting down her fork and switching to coffee, I ate everything on my plate.

"You have such a big appetite!" Christina marveled.

I was mortified. Sure, Christina looked great and had a ton of energy, I told myself, but what kind of grown woman orders pancakes shaped like Mickey Mouse?

Two weekends later my friend Elizabeth and her husband Darren came to meet us for dinner in a nearby town. I like Darren, but he's definitely a guy's guy—business school, basketball, blunt conversation. We went for Italian food in a small-town restaurant with big plastic menus. I ate everything on my plate and then scooped up some of Neil's food when he offered me a taste of his pasta. Darren looked at me like I was from another planet and made some comment about how in his experience, it was the husband who ate off his wife's plate. He didn't mean to embarrass me; he was just being honest. But once more I was humiliated. Again, someone was pointing out my lack of portion control. I thought about his comment over the next several days and began to realize that if generally preoccupied Darren noticed my eating habits and thought them so unusual, maybe I really did have a problem.

That's when it began to hit me that the concept of truthfulness—discussed by my yoga teachers in class, and covered in my yoga philosophy books—applied not just to what came out of my mouth but also to what I put into it. My teacher in New York, an artist named Ruth who taught at the Jivamukti Yoga Center, always opened her classes with a discussion of yoga philosophy. We'd sit on multicolored Mexican blankets with our legs crossed and our hands earnestly placed palms up on our knees or in prayer position at our chest while she offered her thoughts. According to Ruth, all of us—not just me and the other young and just-starting-out women in class, but our celebrity classmates as well—face similar kinds of moral and emotional challenges in life. There's no single teaching that can take away all of our problems, she would say—no simple lesson that can act as a magic salve for all emotional wounds. But the Sutras teach that truthfulness is essential for resolving any kind of problem that may come our way. Ruth challenged us to become more genuine with ourselves and to start living our lives more authentically.

I'd taken what she said seriously; examining my life through the lens of truthfulness had led me to realize that my relationship with my parents was beyond repair. But there *was* something I wasn't being honest with myself about, something that was right on the surface for everyone around me to see—how much I was eating. I thought of my mother, making herself sick with food. I didn't want diabetes in my future. Forget about being a certain size; more than anything, I wanted to feel comfortable in my own skin again, healthy and strong like I'd felt on that mountaintop in Nepal. It was time to apply the concept of truthfulness to my diet. Could practicing *satya* help me get thin? At forty pounds overweight, it was worth a try.

Excuses, Excuses

During that time, when it came to my body, I made every excuse in the book. I tried to never step on a scale, but when I did, I rationalized away my weight gain. Again and again I told myself lies—about what I was eating and what was happening to my body. In this I wasn't alone.

Most overeaters aren't truthful with themselves. For example, we don't cook at home regularly but instead go out to eat or do takeout, deceiving ourselves about how much oil, saturated fat, and other unhealthy ingredients may be going into our meal—a subconscious way of relinquishing control of our bodies to strangers who work in restaurant kitchens. It breaks my heart to have lunch with an overweight friend at her regular spot—a supposedly healthy salad place—where they fill her bowl with whatever high-calorie ingredients she points to: cheese, buttery croutons, oily dressing. She *thinks* she's making a healthy dietetic choice—a salad!—and doesn't understand why she's not losing weight. Then there's my new-mom friend in New York who has a bran muffin every morning but *can't understand* why she isn't dropping the last of her baby weight. Likewise, when we do gain weight, we blame it on water retention, or premenstrual bloating, or the thickness of our pajamas, or the time of day we get on the scale. We tell ourselves that we hate being fat but depend on the weight to help protect us from rejection, from the fear of failure— because if we're still unhappy when we're thin, then what?

The first step on *my* road to truthfulness—and to getting thin—was understanding *why* I was overeating and seeing the link between my caloric intake and the physical abuse I'd suffered as a child. Like so many overweight people, I'd put on body armor to protect myself against what felt like an emotionally unsafe world.

The Myth of the Feminist French Fry

One of the excuses I used to tell myself in college was that a *real* feminist wouldn't care about her weight. It wasn't until I got to Nepal and lost weight by eating a vegetarian diet and doing all that hiking that I realized how fantastic it feels to be thin and, more important, healthy. For the first time in my life, trekking through Nepal on that independent study, I was alone—not lonely in the familiar eat-a-bowl-of-pistachio-nuts-before-bed-while-reading-novels-and-listening-to-The-Smiths kind of way but in the I-am-a-kickass-woman-climbing-mountains-singing-musical-scores-and-sleeping-in-teahouses-while-speaking-Nepalese kind of way. I didn't even realize how much weight I was losing.

But when I left Nepal, I realized that this much-lighter me was, shockingly enough, *still a feminist.* In other words, *I did not have to be fat to be a feminist.* Amazing what a liberal arts education and a semester abroad in a developing country will teach you. Now that I'm both a card-carrying feminist and a five-minute-headstand-doing yogi, I realize that, if anything, being at a healthy weight (and no longer depressed) makes me *more* of a capable woman and feminist, not less.

Living in the country, surrounded by the calming Berkshire hills and the houses with their peeling paint, the dairy cows grazing down the road, I found the mental space to look inward, to think about how I was raised to deal with food, and how these were patterns I needed to change. I started doing the inner psychological work necessary to see myself as others in my life saw me—as a loving and lovable person. That was the first layer of truthfulness.

But, however necessary, it was just the first step.

〜

Huffing and Puffing on Mount Mohonk

Overindulging in fatty foods wasn't my only problem. Another way I wasn't being truthful with myself had to do with how much exercise I was getting (or, rather, *not* getting) and, the flip side of the caloric equation—portion control.

The third visitor during our summer in the country was Leigh. We'd been housemates in Madison. Like me, Leigh had moved to New York after graduation. A political activist, line cook, and artist, of all my girlfriends, Leigh was the last to care about conforming to a skinny beauty ideal. She took the train up one August weekend with plans to go on a day hike and then out for a special dinner before driving back to our house. On the hike, I huffed and puffed on the easy-enough trail and was uncomfortable in what had previously been my loosest pair of pants. I was surprised; I still thought of myself as an adept hiker, though it had been years since my time in Nepal.

The more we lead a life of honesty, the more we will see the results.

—Sri Swami Satchidananda

The problem was the new weight hanging on me. I felt each of those extra pounds I carried up the trail. With Neil up ahead, I mentioned something to Leigh—gingerly and with a lot of embarrassment—about my increasing weight. She'd noticed the change in me, too—I'd been thinner back in Madison—and wasn't surprised or made uncomfortable by my comment. I think she was waiting for me to say something, to open up to her. Leigh made me feel like it was okay to talk about what was going on with me.

After the hike, we went out for dinner at a restaurant with a lodge-like interior and a New American cuisine menu. Neil managed the order, playing the part of a good host, but I felt something was off. There were several appetizers on the table and an entrée for each of us, plus dessert. Despite the comment I'd made earlier to Leigh about my weight, Neil and I stuffed ourselves. Leigh ate like a typical foodie, tasting everything, but not overdoing it on any one dish. I, on the other hand, left the table feeling sick—sick to my stomach and sick of living my life this way.

On our second and last night together, Leigh cooked for us, grilling vegetables we'd picked up from a local farm and serving them with soba noodles in a delicious, low-calorie sauce. The yellows, oranges, and greens of the vegetables popped off the plate. We spread a blanket outside on the grass, watched the sunset, and ate the light and perfect summer meal. *This* was how I needed to eat if I wanted to lose weight and be able to hike Mount Mohonk without struggling to catch my breath. I finally got it.

Leigh's Grilled (or Roasted) Vegetables

Cut green or red peppers, zucchini, carrots, asparagus stalks, and onions, in thick slices, toss with a light sprinkling of extra virgin olive oil, and place on skewers. Feel free to experiment with vegetable choices. Sprinkle with sea salt and spread on a grill, or in a 450-degree oven. Cook until slightly golden—just a few minutes. Squeeze a lemon over the veggies and serve a generous portion with a modest side of soba noodles or brown rice, or another whole grain of your choice. For a light low-calorie sauce, prepare a simple mustard vinaigrette with Dijon mustard, balsamic vinegar, and a little bit of olive oil. Add chopped cucumber and tomato; serve warm or cool.

Top Six Signs You Are Eating Too Much

1. Your "fat" clothes have become your favorite clothes. "Stretchy" is the new black.

2. No matter how big the restaurant portion size, you have no problem eating everything on your plate. The saying "Her eyes are bigger than her stomach"? Well, you have the opposite problem.

3. The number on the scale keeps going up, no matter how many times a week you go to the gym. It can't all be muscle weight . . .

4. You prefer eating out with your heavier friends so you don't feel badly about what you're ordering.

5. You tell yourself that a muffin or bagel in the morning is perfectly healthy—just "a little something" for breakfast.

6. You decide your scale must be broken and throw it in the garbage.

Leigh wasn't just a sensible eater; though far from an exercise fanatic, she also loved a good walk. I did too, but I'd gotten out of the habit of walking regularly during my depression. The next morning, she suggested we take a walk through the country roads that wound through town before she caught her train home. We walked past the "downtown"— meaning the post office, bank, and convenience store where we bought our newspaper and milk—beyond the houses off Main Street, and out to one of the farms on the far end of town. An older man chopping firewood waved to us from his yard. We spotted deer along the way and noticed all the different shades of green in the hills. On that walk, I felt the peace I'd often felt in yoga class. I realized how easy it would be to walk the same route—which took no more than fifty minutes—most days.

Wake Up and Smell the Green Tea

The Monday morning after Leigh's visit, I rolled out my yoga mat as usual. The physical poses alone weren't going to help me lose all that excess weight, but I sensed that practicing the series of ancient stretches could connect me to something deeper that would eventually be the key to my slimming salvation. It was tempting to give myself a hard time—how could I have let things get this bad? But beating myself up wouldn't help. What I needed to do was start fresh, re-evaluating what I ate and how I moved from the moment I woke up in the morning until I went to bed at night. In yoga class—back in New York, and in Mexico—I'd felt clean and light and healthy. Could I find a way to eat that well and move my body consistently in my everyday life?

"Can We Please Stop and Get Some Fruit?"

Another friend of mine, Jackie, helped me see that I could. Jackie is originally from California, and we met while she was attending grad school. Growing up, Jackie had always been at a healthy weight, but she lost an additional ten pounds walking all over New York, exploring the city. (When I say walking all over the city, I'm not exaggerating. One spring Jackie worked as an intern at a public elementary school in Harlem. A couple of times a week she would walk from NYU in the Village to her school all the way uptown, and then back down again at the end of the day to her apartment in Chelsea—more than an hour and a half *each* way at a very brisk pace.)

Jackie also came to visit us that summer, and remembering how much she loved walking—and how great she looked as a result—gave me new inspiration to take my daily country walks. But I learned another enlightening lesson from Jackie, too. One of the first questions she asked after she arrived—almost before "How are you?" and "Where's the bathroom?"—was whether we had any fruit in the house. The answer, sadly, was not really. Maybe we had a banana or two, or an orange. But Jackie wanted more than that. She asked us to drive her to the local food co-op where she piled a shopping bag full of pineapple, apples, grapes, melon, and summer fruits.

Back at home, she carved into the pineapple, lopping off the top and bottom, and then slicing through the center to get to the sweet fruit meat inside—something I didn't know how to do (pineapples had always intimidated me with their prickly exteriors). She made a heaping bowl of fruit salad that we immediately started to snack on, and we used it as a basis for breakfast all weekend long.

Fruit! Before Jackie's visit I'd never realized how filling and delicious fruit could be, or that a pineapple could become a serious part of my health regimen. From Jackie's example I learned to always, always have fruit in the house—and to make fruit my go-to snack when hunger strikes. Soon I started having a bowl of pineapple for breakfast every morning. From Leigh and Jackie I now had two effective ideas for how to get started moving my body and changing my diet. Just adding a forty-five to sixty-minute walk each day and replacing my less-healthful snacks with fruit, and I was already on my way to shedding weight.

Jackie's Fruit Salad

Cut up thick slices of pineapple, apple, melon, and banana, adding a handful of grapes or whatever seasonal fruits you like, such as strawberries. Combine in a large mixing or salad bowl. Keep in the fridge at all times for easy access; fruit can be one of the first things you reach for when you're hungry. The mixture of the flavors creates a natural sauce.

Jessica's New Favorite Breakfast

1/3 of a pineapple

1 banana

1/4 cup organic low-fat plain or vanilla yogurt

A sprinkling of almonds (no more than 6 or 8 when trying to lose weight)

Why Pineapple Can Help You Lose Weight

Recently I asked Marion Nestle, a renowned nutrition expert and professor at New York University, to explain why pineapple might have helped me lose weight. "Pineapple has a lot of water along with its calories, and that fills you up," Nestle told me. "Any fruit should do that." Unlike processed cereals or bread products, fruits have low caloric density—meaning you can eat more of them and still keep your calories down. So make the switch to a big bowl of your favorite fruits for breakfast or a mid-morning meal.

I became so addicted to this incredibly filling and satisfying breakfast that now friends make sure to buy pineapple for me before I come to visit. If you start eating this breakfast on a regular basis, prepare to take questions from grocery store cashiers about your piña colada fixation.

How to Cut a Pineapple

I promise—it's not as complicated as it looks. Chop off the top and bottom of the pineapple with a kitchen knife, and then slice horizontally into the middle of the fruit, cutting it in half. Next, cut away at the prickly outside. With what's left, slice into chunks away from the small hard core, and then cut into smaller bite-size pieces.

A Few Notes about Yogurt

Avoid yogurt that contains "fruit." These are loaded with sugar and, almost always, with artificial ingredients. According to Marion Nestle, the closer we stick to plain, unflavored yogurt, the better off we'll be, even though she admits in her fantastic book, *What to Eat,* that "unflavored yogurt is an acquired taste." She suggests adding your own sugar or honey; no matter what, you'll add less than the yogurt companies do. I like to use just a little vanilla low-fat yogurt with live bacteria; the bacteria, or yogurt cultures, are what makes this something more than just a sweet dessert. Still, use sparingly.

The ability to be honest in communication with sensitivity, without hurting others, without telling lies, and with the necessary reflection requires a very refined state of being. Such persons cannot make mistakes in their actions.

—T. K. V. Desikachar

Pastry Confessions

Even after you've lost weight, practicing *satya* will come in handy when it comes to maintaining. Though he didn't have nearly as much to shed as I did, my husband Neil couldn't help but lose weight once we started eating differently. He went from a medium-sized five-foot-ten man with a developing paunch to a slim and lithe 140-pound hottie—and this without much actual yoga practice. A certified workaholic professor, Neil doesn't set aside much time for yoga. There are months when he doesn't make it to class, when the best he can do is fall into a restorative pose on the living room floor. But changing his eating and exercise habits—becoming a vegetarian for starters (more on that later), walking around the neighborhood rather than driving, doing push-ups while watching television, and adding in the occasional weekend hike or jog—has kept Neil skinny and energetic into his late thirties. As his guy friends enter early middle age and start gaining weight and potbellies, and Neil keeps getting slimmer and younger-looking, the health benefits of these yogic eating and living habits have become more and more obvious.

But, like many people, Neil has a sweet tooth. (Sweets have never been my thing—give me a toasted bagel with cream cheese and tomato over cake for breakfast any day—but Neil craves sugar in the mornings to go with his coffee.) When he indulges and treats himself to a pastry once or twice a week, he invariably reports back to me that evening about his snack. For a long time, I teased him—for both the morning indulgence and the need to confess. After all, I'm his wife, not his mother. It's not really my business what he eats for breakfast, is it? And then I realized that Neil's pastry confessions are his way of living truthfully. We all need to report to someone, to be accountable for our health and daily habits.

Neil and I are now comfortable enough with each other to have frank check-ins about how we're doing with our eating and exercise. I trust that, when I ask him to, Neil will be able to give me an honest assessment of how I'm doing. It's a lot less painful to hear you need to lose a couple pounds than to wait until it's a matter of twenty or fifty. Your truthtelling partner doesn't have to be your romantic interest; I can understand why this might not seem like an appealing way to go. Maybe it's a friend or coworker or sibling, or even a therapist—but being accountable to someone, and coming clean about what you're eating, is an important part of living truthfully.

Top Five Signs You Need to Take a Hike

1. Walking from your parking space to the office is your most regular workout.

2. Your sports bra and sneakers are collecting dust in your closet.

3. The last time you communed with nature, you were at sleep-away camp.

4. Just reading about Jackie's walks through Manhattan made you tired.

5. Your dog has given up asking for anything more than a stroll around the block. And she's starting to look a little pudgy, too.

On the Mat

With the last of our summer houseguests on their way back to the city, determined to face the truth at last, I stepped on the scale and finally took in what it said: 150 pounds. Okay, maybe 152. Much too much for my petite frame. (For many women, 150 may be a perfectly healthy weight—it all depends on height, frame, age, etc. But any medical professional would have taken a look at me and advised me to lose weight.) It could have been worse, but I also knew it could have been a lot better. So I returned to the yoga philosophy books I'd started studying and rededicated myself to yoga practice and to daily walks through the country roads that wound around our house. Once a week I drove forty-five minutes to take a yoga class in another town. There, and at home, I worked on the same basic poses I'd always practiced but this time with a new sense of purpose, holding the postures more deeply and for longer chunks of time.

Any yoga pose takes concentration and dedication. The more you focus on a given pose and lengthen the time spent in it, the more challenging that pose becomes; even those that look simple at first glance can become a workout. I found that a good place to start practicing truthfulness is in the basic standing pose illustrated at the start of this chapter, mountain pose. It's said that an advanced yogi can stand in mountain pose for many minutes and drip sweat from the hard work and attention needed to remain still with complete attention and commitment. For now, practice standing on your own two feet with solidity and a flowing and free breath. Get in touch with your personal truths. Why are you unhappy? Why are you overweight? Not to get too Southern California on you but see if you can stand firm in the knowledge of who you are, and who you hope to become.

Being honest and confronting old demons and engrained eating habits are the first steps toward getting enlightened. But clearly, I also needed to eat less. Much less. The books I was studying emphasized the importance of moderation. I knew I needed to start with what I was putting in my mouth.

4

moderation
(*brahmacarya*)

THE HALF-EMPTY STOMACH

(SELF-RESTRAINT,
SELF-CONTROL, MODERATION)

SUTRA II.38: *BRAHMACARYAPRATISTHAYAM
VIRYALABHAH*

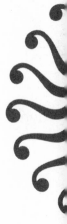

When the *sadhaka* [seeker] is firmly established in continence, knowledge, vigour, valour, and energy flow to him.

—B. K. S. Iyengar

Don't Eat Too Much

According to the yogic tradition, a balanced life is characterized by moderation in all things. The Sanskrit term for moderation in diet is *mitahara*. For some people, radical lifestyles are the goal—the monk, the priest, the Olympic athlete, the businessperson or political campaign worker who works eighty-hour weeks. For the yogi, living a life of moderation is the most radical step of all. But how do you get there when it comes to food?

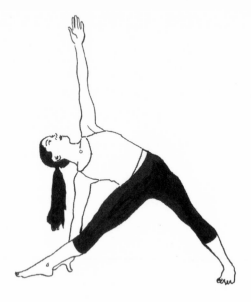

Begin the pose by standing with your legs wide apart. Turn your right leg out so that your right foot is perpendicular with your left heel. Bending from your hip socket, extend your torso and right arm out toward the right side of the room. Place your right hand on your right leg below your knee, on a yoga block placed behind your right leg, or on the floor. Keep your left hand on your left hip and dynamically turn your chest and hips to the left. Lift and open your chest. Raise your left arm straight up and look up at your hand, or—if this bothers your neck—directly in front of you. Repeat on the other side. As you work on the give and take between your legs, torso, and arms in this pose, stand firm in your commitment to doing all things in moderation, including eating.

At its best, moderation produces the highest individual vitality. . . . Nothing is wasted by us if we seek to develop moderation in all things. Too much of anything brings problems. Too little may be inadequate.

—T. K. V. Desikachar

The philosophical underpinnings of moderation are drawn from the yoga sutra on *brahmacarya*, or celibacy and continence. Following in the yogic path, the Sutras say, means figuring out how to control and channel our sexual and sensual energies. Moderation is a virtue because it's the opposite of gluttony; rather than needing to fulfill every desire to the maximum, be content with smaller servings of pleasure. This isn't necessarily about taking a vow of chastity. Moderation, at its best, is about living in the moment, being okay with what you have right now, about seeing the pineapple bowl as half full rather than half empty. Living this way, when it comes to food and material possessions, teaches us to generally appreciate where we are in life.

Be Here Now

I was first introduced to the concept of *brahmacarya,* and the corollary principle of moderation, through the teachings of a modern-day yoga philosopher named Ram Dass. While the ideas sounded good in theory, I doubted my ability to put them into practice. How could I give up my constant desire for more, in eating or in any other area of my life?

Dass discusses *brahmacarya,* among other yogic concepts, in a book titled *Be Here Now,* a handbook and introduction to all things groovy and yogic. Dass, I soon realized, wasn't an Indian-born philosopher but a major hippie guru born and bred in the West. Way back when, he'd been a young psychology professor at Harvard known as Richard Alpert. At Harvard, Alpert met Timothy Leary, a promoter of psychedelic experience, and together they and their growing band of followers started tuning in and dropping out. Alpert then traveled to India, where he came to realize that true consciousness comes not from adding drugs to the biochemical mix but from stripping away everything that can cloud consciousness—be it drugs, food, materialism, or having a big ego. Though Dass was old enough to be my father, or even grandfather, I related to him and his journey and was moved by the loving way in which he'd written about the relationship he had with his guru, a simply robed Indian man named Neem Karoli Baba, with devotees hailing from all over the globe.

In the "Cookbook for a Sacred Life" section of *Be Here Now*, Ram Dass offers some tips for how to live a yogic life. When it comes to diet, he tells his readers simply: "Don't eat too much." No New Age mumbo jumbo there—just good advice. "Eat light, healthy, unadulterated foods which are easily digestible," Dass says, "substituting whole grains, such as brown rice and whole wheat, along with vegetables, some fish, fruit, honey instead of sugar, nuts and dairy products." He advises going light on coffee, tea, and alcohol, too. These were concrete steps I could take.

The Golden Rule of Yogic Eating

Elaborating further, Dass shared the magical formula for eating like a yogi. What a revelation!

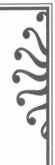

Eat Like a Yogi

After a meal, your stomach should be

1/2 full with food,

1/4 full with water, and

1/4 empty with room for air.

As a child, I'd been taught to eat everything on my plate, whether I was hungry or not. Finishing my dinner meant I was "a big girl" (if only they knew), a good girl—while leaving too much food on my plate was a sign of disobedience and disrespect. I should be grateful for that meatloaf, for those frozen string beans. As a mother, I get it: My parents worked hard to fill my plate, and they wanted me to reap the benefits. They did the best they could. But when we teach children to eat this way, we disable the inner food compasses we're all born with, the little guru of moderation inside each of us that knows when we've had enough.

Even as an adult, though I usually ate less than I did as a kid, I still had the urge to go overboard when it came to portion size. I've already told you how I ate and ate the year I was depressed and going through the painful break with my parents. That was a case of eating to fill an emotional hole. Yet sometimes, immoderation comes from the desire to please others. . . .

A Hanukkah Story

Last holiday season, my husband Neil and I decided to throw a Hanukkah party for our friends and neighbors. We settled on brunch and planned to make latkes, the traditional fried potato pancakes. Latkes are basically the opposite of a health food, but we figured everyone could have a little taste. A small latke, maybe two. A sliver of birthday cake for our son Lucien, who was born the previous Christmas Eve. That was the plan anyway. Neil agreed to do the grocery shopping and to prep the potatoes the afternoon before while I stayed home to take care of the baby.

Neil is a kind and generous guy. When he got to the store he decided to multiply our planned quantities of food for the party by two or three—just in case.

"Sweetie?" I asked, looking through the dozen bags he'd brought home from the supermarket and bagel shop, studying the hefty bill. "How much food did you buy?" Attempting to remain calm, I rummaged through the merchandise: three extra large containers of orange juice, seven cream cheeses, five dozen bagels, and several fields' worth of potatoes.

"We only have fifty people coming," I said. "And a lot of those are babies!"

I'll spare you the details of the argument that followed. Suffice it to say, Neil insisted I was being a scrooge, and I insisted he was over the top. Wanting to make sure nobody would be deprived of a latke, Neil proceeded to fry up 150 of them. I focused on baking a vegan birthday cake, which, given my lack of baking expertise, didn't leave too much time for squabbling.

The next day we woke up to a brilliant white blizzard. About half of our guests couldn't come because of the road conditions. We had a great party anyway—music, kids, latkes, and cake. But we had five times as much food as we needed. Neil solved the problem by sending guests home with a bag of bagels and cream cheese in one hand, and plates of leftover latkes in the other. He worked on cleaning up the kitchen while I put the baby to sleep.

"You were right," Neil said when I came in. "Next year, I'll only make a hundred."

Veggie Chili

Okay, okay, in theory you'd love to eat like a bird, a French woman, a skinny bitch, and a yogi. But, realistically, how can you go about changing your appetite without some drastic measure like gastric bypass surgery? Your hunger's not going to disappear just by reading some yoga philosophy or doing some downward dogs. What you need are practical steps. Implementing moderation in eating is simpler than you'd think: First, you need a few good staple meals, and, second, you need a change in perspective.

Early on in the year I lost forty pounds, Neil and I came across a simple recipe for vegetarian chili. All it involved was opening up some cans of black beans and crushed tomatoes and a jar of salsa, chopping and sautéing some broccoli, heating and serving. When we remembered, we sprinkled in coriander and cumin, but the only necessity was a little sea salt. The chili—cheap, filling, nutritious, warming, and low-calorie—was essential to my weight loss. We ate it several times a week that year. Having a healthy default meal like chili makes it less likely that when you're exhausted and starving at the end of the day, and you can't figure out what to make, you'll do something self-defeating like pick up the phone and order a pizza. This recipe makes a *big* vat of chili—enough for two adults and two young children, or three adults, or two adults plus leftovers for a big lunch the next day.

Neil's Veggie Chili (with thanks to the Moosewood Cookbook series)

1 medium-sized yellow onion, chopped

2 heads broccoli, washed and chopped (enough to make about 2 cups)

1 teaspoon olive oil

1 28-oz. can of crushed organic
   tomatoes

1 16-oz. can of salsa

2 15-oz. cans of organic black beans* or 3 1/2 cups cooked beans

2 teaspoons sea salt

1 teaspoon cumin

1 teaspoon coriander

Put oil in a pot on medium heat. When hot, add onions, cumin, and coriander. Cook for 2 minutes or until onion gets soft. Add broccoli and salt and cook for 2 minutes more, stirring frequently. Add tomatoes, salsa, and black beans, and stir. Cook on medium-low heat for 10 minutes, stirring occasionally. The broccoli should cook through but not get overly soft. Add additional salt to taste. Serve with a modest sprinkling of part-skim organic mozzarella cheese.

*A note on beans: For years now, I'd heard that homemade beans are easy to make, cheaper, and more environmentally friendly (no excess packaging) than canned, and much more delicious. But you *do* have to plan ahead when making beans at home, as they have to be soaked for several hours before cooking. So I resisted. Finally, a friend convinced me to try them. They were delicious—so much better than canned—and the process wasn't anywhere near as time-consuming as I'd imagined. All you need to do is buy loose beans (of any sort—you can start with black and go from there), rinse them, put them in a pot with a few inches of water covering them, bring to a boil, then turn off the heat for about two hours while the beans soak. Then simmer them in the water remaining in the pot, adding more as necessary, for about fifteen minutes to half an hour—or however long it takes them to become tender—before serving. Add a pinch of sea salt to taste. Make a big batch and stick the leftovers in the refrigerator (or drain and freeze) for easy reheating.

But you also need a perspective shift. Like I said, for months we ate the chili all the time—nothing tasted so good. While cutting calories during the day and eliminating late-night snacking was difficult, I was comforted by the thought of sitting down to a thoroughly satisfying bowl of chili sometime in the near future. When we first started eating veggie chili, Neil would dish up the bowls and serve them with a slice or two of toasted whole-wheat bread and a sprinkling of cheese. We'd scoop the toast into the chili, making miniature black bean sandwiches. Super tasty and good. For seconds, we'd refill our bowls halfway, sometimes all the way. Then one day we left a bag of groceries behind at the store. Since we were living twenty-five minutes away from the nearest supermarket, we had our chili sans toast. We thought it would be a deprivation—that dinner just wouldn't be the same, that we might have to forage for nuts and berries on the road outside our house, make an emergency run into town for ice cream sundaes . . . To our shock, the chili was perfectly satisfying on its own.

We nixed the bread permanently—and I lost more weight within days. (Since that discovery, putting all bread products, including my beloved bagels, in the "once in a blue moon" category has helped me keep the weight off these past seven years.) Anyway, there we were, for months, happily eating our chili without toast. And then one day, we forgot the cheese. Again, we realized that the chili tasted good without the cheese on top! Finally, I figured out that if I didn't refill my bowl for seconds, I could still be perfectly content and get a good night's sleep (my big fear about limiting portions at dinner). I mean, duh! But I'd grown up using that filled-up-with-food feeling as a kind of comfort, an emotional crutch, especially in the evening and before bed. To see that one-fourth air left in my stomach could actually be a pleasant sensation rather than a source of distress was a big shift in my thinking. Slowly but surely, my appetite adjusted to this new way of moderate eating, decreasing over the months and years that followed. My craving for healthy foods increased over time, too.

The broader lesson here is that losing weight in a moderate, healthy, and yogic way is a *gradual* process. Start with a good, reasonably low-calorie staple meal, and one day you'll be ready to pare down and lower your caloric intake a little more, and then after a while, more again.

As I started to lose more and more weight, I focused on eating as healthfully as possible and cutting out anything that lacked nutritional value. Dr. Andrew Weil's books were a sensible companion to my yoga books and became my nutritional bibles. No more packaged foods and partially hydrogenated oils, Weil insisted; no more diet sodas. Instead, I ate lots of fruits and vegetables, along with plenty of lentils. Out went white-flour breads and pastas and in came whole grains like brown rice, quinoa, and spelt, or whole-wheat tortillas. (No, I didn't know what quinoa was either. It's a delicious whole grain that tastes a little like couscous, only heartier, and it's a good source of protein. It's easy to make—put equal parts quinoa and water into a pot and then simmer until the water has been absorbed, about ten to twelve minutes.) Occasionally, we'd have brown rice pasta with broccoli and tomato sauce—making sure that our (small) bowls were filled with two-thirds broccoli, one-third pasta.

Our favorite dinners were chili or vegetarian burritos. Once or twice a week we'd have a yam with a side of sautéed kale. Edamame, the soybean pods on the menu at Japanese restaurants, became a new favorite snack. We cooked lots of tofu, too, limiting the amount of oil we used.

And guess what? The pounds started coming off. Between changing my diet and adding cardio to my yoga (not just the walking, but some gym time, too, which I'll write more about in the next chapter), by the end of our year in the Berkshires I'd lost forty pounds.

Recipe for a Moderate Meal

- Stay hydrated so you don't confuse thirst for hunger.

- Eat mindfully. Concentrate on your food, the colors and textures and tastes in each bite. Eat slowly so your body has time to digest the food and your head can register that "full enough" feeling.

- At some point in the meal—likely sooner than you'd imagine—a quiet voice inside will raise the thought that maybe you've had enough. You might want to resist the thought. Instead, experiment with listening to it.

- Take one last small bite, savor it, and then end your meal. Remember, you can always have something else (a piece of fruit, say) later on. It's okay to be a little hungry!

That May I turned thirty, and Neil and I prepared to leave upstate New York for Los Angeles, where he'd taken a new job and I'd enrolled in a more in-depth yoga teacher–training program. We had a small, idyllic wedding on the grass outside our rented house. Friends came from across the country to help us celebrate. Their eyes widened—I saw a dozen double takes that weekend—to see me changed so much for the better. It wasn't just the weight loss they were struck by; my spirit had lightened, too. Along with the weight, the cloud of depression that had hovered over me off and on throughout my life had finally lifted.

Hoping for a Baby

But, sometimes, just as we're over one hilltop, another appears in the distance. Not long after we got married, Neil and I started trying to have a baby.

I'd wanted to be a mother ever since I was a teenager. My maternal fantasy came to me whole, like a vision: My dream was to be a clog-wearing, baby-toting, milk-producing, sleep-deprived and dirty-haired, deliriously happy earth mother. I was greedy and wanted it all—the station wagon with the dog in the back, the camping trips in the mountains, the husband who helped out and cooked dinner and took the baby on Saturdays, the house with a porch. Most of all, I just wanted the child part of the equation, someone to read books to in the mornings before naptime and take for walks in the woods. I craved the opportunity to create a familial tie based on good feelings and a healthy love, to envelop my baby in safety and comfort, and let her explore the world with confidence.

We started trying in L.A. Each month I was sure I was pregnant—and then my period came. It took us many months to make a pregnancy happen, and when that pregnancy ended in a miscarriage, I grieved deeply. My fantasizing turned to hard-core coveting and envy. Moms were everywhere, in streets and parks and restaurants and bookstores, exhausted and euphoric, and so were their trade accessories I coveted with the full force of greed and wanting, the symbols and signs of the life I couldn't yet have: the overpriced strollers, the "native carrier" baby slings, the plastic bags loaded with secondhand clothes my friends promised to save for me, the wooden toys imported from Germany, the rocking chairs and gliders and hipster kid decals for my would-be nursery walls. What's more, acquaintances and friends were getting pregnant right and left. Every time I checked my e-mail it seemed like there was a new announcement waiting for me—some friends had two or even three babies during the years I longed for a child. Baby shower invitations came in the mail and sent me to bed crying or onto the couch to watch mindless television for the rest of the night. I refused to shop for baby gifts or attend baby showers and would send gift certificates and L.L. Bean tote bags instead.

Mostly I tried to be patient, to take cleansing breaths and find comfort in my yoga practice. To be honest, I reveled in being thin—the one "advantage" of not being pregnant, in my mind. Sometimes, I clung to my hard-won thinness too tightly. For a few months, stressed and sad, I got too skinny.

At first, Neil and I decided against going down the medical route after an initial bad experience with infertility drugs. We applied for an international adoption and began a process that unexpectedly took years rather than months. And then, after one too many waiting-list difficulties and disappointments, as my thirty-fifth birthday approached, I felt we couldn't—*I* couldn't—wait even one month more. We decided to try a round of in vitro fertilization and were indescribably lucky: I became pregnant with my son Lucien on our first attempt.

A happy ending, one for which I daily thank God, the universe, and our infertility clinic. Needless to say, I wouldn't wish miscarriage or infertility on anyone, but those years of waiting and wanting and disappointment taught me something valuable. Among the other virtues discussed in the Yoga Sutras are the concepts of non-hoarding, non-stealing, and non-coveting. Like moderation, these themes certainly apply to body and weight issues. It's important to set goals for yourself but don't waste your time and energy coveting your neighbor's body. Yet these concepts relate to so much more as well.

During the years I struggled with infertility, I learned how to live—how to be okay—despite what I was missing, despite my feeling that I *needed* a child. I never did make it past the feeling that I had to become a mom one way or another, but on my good days at least, I did make the most of the seemingly endless time before me. I wrote and taught and studied yoga. I hung out and had adventures with my husband. I cried with him, too. We grew closer. I made new friends and built supportive and nurturing relationships. I learned to take care of myself. Although my life didn't feel complete without a child, I came to understand that maybe, just maybe, I could wake up on any given morning and drink my cup of coffee and tend to my e-mails, hand in my writing assignments, teach my writing classes, go for a long walk, practice my yoga poses, clean the apartment, empty the dishwasher. For that day, anyway, I would be okay.

Salem

While we waited for a baby to enter our lives, we decided to get a dog. Who would have thought a dog could teach you lessons about yogic eating and living? But sometimes, as it turns out, the guru wears fur. One freezing February morning, back when we were living on the East Coast, Neil and I drove to an animal shelter. There she was—the third member of our family. Salem, as we named her on the ride home, was a small, scared thing, with a white coat and brown and black spots. She was fourteen weeks old and looked absolutely miserable in the corner of her crate. The attached yellow index card said she was a beagle/pointer mix, driven up from a farm where she'd been found and fostered down south. A staff member scooped her out of her crate and placed her in my arms.

"She's the one," I told Neil. This wasn't our first dog-scouting visit, but it was the first time we'd been introduced to a dog that felt like ours. She was cute, cuddly, curious, and slightly neurotic. The family resemblance was immediately noted. We took her outside and she squatted down and did her business, a bright yellow spot tunneling through the snow, creating a permanent opening in our hearts, no matter the piles of dog hair that would be shed in the years to come, ridiculously early morning walks demanded, anti-bark dog collars bought and eaten through, reams of tennis balls destroyed, and dog "hotel" bills paid when we dared to vacation without her.

Not to get too *Marley and Me*, but Salem enrolled us in a multi-year course in life lessons, doggie style. Selfless love and devotion were perennial subjects on the syllabus. So were long daily exercise walks, no matter how busy, tired, sick, or otherwise occupied we believed ourselves to be. Another thing we noticed right away about Salem was her natural tendency toward moderation in eating.

Salem eats when she's hungry, as many as two or three bowls at a time, and won't so much as snack when she's not. At first, we worried when she would go a day or two without eating. Neil would fuss over her, pouring wet canned food on top of her organic dry food. He even called the veterinarian a couple of times to find out what to do if she wouldn't eat. Of course, eventually she would. After a year or so, we figured out that she would always take in enough calories to keep her energy up and her BMI (body mass index) down. Some days this meant a bowl or two of food, some days, not so much as a bite. It all depended on her activity level. After a long afternoon off-leash hike, she's ravenous. On inside days when she's mostly napped as I work at the computer, she might not touch her food once. She eats more when she exercises, less when she doesn't. When it comes to yogic eating, Salem's a natural.

Lessons from Salem

1. Some days are three-bowl days; others, all you need is a little nibble or nosh. Most days, it's nice to be a moderate eater. Don't eat just because you think you're supposed to (the ding-it's-dinnertime mentality), and likewise, don't starve yourself on days—and times of life, like pregnancy—when you truly do need extra calories.

2. The dog park is *always* a good idea. While Salem will, on occasion, turn down a bowl of food, she'll never refuse a run around the dog park. She can *always* find a second, third, or fourth wind. There'll be time for a nap later

on. Emulate Salem and embrace the joy and freedom in moving your body. Find the pleasure in it. Rather than seeing daily walks or workouts as a chore, view them in a new light, as the one time of day when you have the luxury of being totally tuned in to yourself and focused on you.

3. Never turn down a cuddle. Looking back to my adolescent nights with a book and a bowl of pistachio nuts, I realize now that what I needed wasn't food but love. Touch is a tonic, and the best medicine for a bad day. Massage, cuddles, partner yoga—trading friendly touch can lessen your desire to eat more than you need, since sometimes those cravings aren't for food but for connection. You don't need a significant other to take advantage of the benefits of touch, either. Snuggle with an animal friend—or volunteer at an animal shelter if you don't have a pet. Check out massage therapy schools in your area, where student massages often come cheap, for as little as $18 for a forty-five-minute session.

All Done

We were blessed. A few years after Salem came to live with us, our son Lucien was born, and another moderate eater joined our household. Believe me, this boy isn't one to turn down a warm breast or a bowl of baby cereal mixed with banana slices. These days, at twelve months old, he's all over his brown rice, avocado and tofu, lentil soup, apple and pear chunks, and pieces of rice cake with spinach hummus. Still, as hungry as he gets, as much as he loves his milk and solids, when he's done, he's done. He has his fill and then turns his head from the breast or bottle or bowl, ready for the next big thing—his pile of board books, an adventurous crawl around the house, or giggling at the antics of his naughty doggie Salem. If we tune in to his signals, they're unmistakable, and have been since he started on solids at six months. "I'm done, Mommy and Daddy," he says with his eyes and pursed lips, and with the way he drops the spoon and looks around the room, pushing his bowl away.

In working toward moderation and non-hoarding in our eating habits, what a blessing it would be if we could all rediscover the naturalness with which Salem and Lucien (and some humans, too) balance the pleasures of satisfying an appetite with the good feeling—and good health—that comes with finding an equilibrium between energy in and energy out.

Chili, my standby meal for years, is no longer in such heavy rotation at our house; I lost the taste for it during my pregnancy. After chili, our new staple became vegetable and black bean burritos with whole-wheat tortillas and some slices of avocado, with vegetables of all sorts and combinations— zucchini, broccoli, mushrooms, chard, green beans. These days we've switched to a vegan stir-fry with whatever vegetables look good (local and organic) at our farmers' market—in the summer, multicolored zucchini, kale, garlic scapes, cherry tomatoes, served with brown rice and tofu, or with quinoa and chickpeas. Come fall, we switch to a simpler version with tofu and broccoli and carrots. The meal is cheap, quick to prepare, healthy, and satisfying, and there are usually leftovers for lunch. (Some practitioners of Ayurveda, the traditional Indian science of health and healing, say that leftovers don't have much *prana*, or life force, so I used to avoid them. But lately, with a baby and writing deadlines and teaching responsibilities and a mortgage, I'm grateful to reheat last night's meal and have something quick and easy to eat while I feed Lucien his lunch. These days I'll make a big vat of brown rice and keep it in the fridge, reheating portions of it in the microwave as I prepare meals.)

Signs You're Eating Too Much

1. You feel full after a meal. If you feel stuffed, you've eaten too much. Leave 1/4 space for air!
2. You feel tired after eating. Food should leave you energetic, not sleepy.
3. You can't wait for the moment after dinner when you change from real clothes to sweats.

Getting Started: Practical Tips for Moderate Eating

1. Start a food diary with the goal of becoming more aware of what you are eating, and how the food makes you feel. Which foods make you feel good after you eat them? Which leave you feeling tired, heavy, or bloated?

2. Change your diet? Change your life.

    Start experimenting by adding more fresh vegetables, legumes, fruits, and whole grains into your meal plan and decreasing the amount of meat, white flours, and junky snack foods. Eat as few processed foods as possible. No hydrogenated oils! (Check the package before you buy to find out what you're eating. If you don't know what the chemicals listed in the ingredients list are, then it's probably not a good idea to eat them. Try to avoid the inside aisles of the supermarket.)

    Slow down when you eat. Don't eat standing up, in the car, or on the run. Sit at a table, even for just a few minutes. Listen to your body for clues as to when you're full; chew slowly and give yourself ten or twenty minutes for the food to sink in before helping yourself to seconds. End meals before feeling completely stuffed, and breathe through the anxiety you feel on leaving the table with that one-fourth of empty space. If you need something sweet, have fruit or a super-small rather than super-sized square of organic dark chocolate. (The fair trade kind makes you feel especially good.)

Drink water. Lots of it—more than you think. In the morning, before meals, and before bed. Chamomile tea is a nice way to stay hydrated, too. Drink it warm in the cold months, or, in the summer, add a tea bag to a pitcher of cold water and ice cubes and make a no-calorie alternative to sugary iced tea.

3. Take a hike.

Begin a moderate daily exercise routine. Stretch your body and spirit with yoga—using the poses at the start of each chapter in this book (practice them in order) and a class in your neighborhood. Do something else, too: Start walking, jogging, playing ball with your dog or kids in your local park. Turn up the music and dance around your bedroom in your pajamas. Do some kind of movement every day. Rather than worry about not having the time, spend that worry time exercising. Can you find twenty minutes a day? Thirty? An hour? Take the stairs instead of the elevator; ride public transportation rather than driving (you'll save money on gas and burn calories walking to the bus or train stop). Walk your baby in her stroller rather than sitting in a café. When friends ask you to catch up with them on the weekends, suggest spending Sunday morning together communing with nature in a park or on a hiking trail. Drop all the excuses holding you back: Just pull on some sneakers, grab some water, and go.

Black Bean Burrito

---

2 whole-wheat or spelt tortillas
   (spelt contains many nutrients and is a good source of protein)

any fresh seasonal veggies (I like broccoli, carrots, zucchini, or chard)

1 teaspoon olive oil

1 15-oz. can of organic black beans (or, even better, homemade beans)

avocado slices

hot sauce

a few fresh cilantro leaves

sprinkling of part-skim organic
   cheddar cheese

Wash and chop vegetables; sauté in a pan with olive oil for about 5 minutes, or until tender but not soggy. (Alternately you can steam the veggies.) Drain and heat black beans separately. In another pan, this one nonstick, warm tortillas on low to medium heat—without oil—for a couple of minutes on each side. Serve with sliced avocado, hot sauce, cheese, and some fresh cilantro. Serves two (two and a half if you have a small child around).

Dragon Bowl (à la *The Angelica Home Kitchen cookbook*)

Sauce:

1 1/3 cups organic tahini (made from ground sesame seeds)

1/3 cup low-sodium organic soy sauce

1/3 cup brown rice syrup (a syrup made from brown rice which metabolizes more slowly than simple sugars)

2 tablespoons Dijon mustard

1/3 cup brown rice vinegar

Place all ingredients in a bowl with one tablespoon hot water. Whisk thoroughly, then cover and refrigerate.

Other ingredients:

2 heads of kale or Swiss chard

1 package medium-firm tofu

1/3 cup low-sodium organic soy sauce

1 cup (dry) brown rice

When brown rice is well under way, start a pot with 1 cup of water and add the soy sauce. When this nears a low boil, add the tofu—cut into bite-sized cubes—and reduce heat to a simmer. Meanwhile, wash and chop the kale or Swiss chard. When rice is about 5 minutes from being done, place vegetables in a pot with about half a cup of water, heat, and cover. (The water will steam the vegetables.) When done, drain the vegetables and the tofu. Assemble bowls with rice on the bottom, veggies on top of the rice, tofu on top of the veggies, and 2 tablespoons of the sauce layered over the whole thing. Serves three.

Veggie Stir-Fry

---

any fresh seasonal veggies, enough to make 4 cups uncooked
brown rice

1   block/package medium-firm organic tofu

1   tablespoon mustard

2   tablespoons low-sodium organic soy sauce

1   teaspoon chopped fresh dill or other
    favorite fresh herb

1   teaspoon olive oil

1   tablespoon grape seed oil ⟶ this readily available oil heats up better than olive oil for cooking tofu and has a neutral flavor

Cook one cup of dry brown rice (use twice as much water as rice; bring to a boil; then reduce heat to low and simmer). After it has been cooking for about 20 minutes, put grape seed oil in a nonstick pan and heat on medium heat. Cut the tofu into bite-sized cubes and place in a pan, stirring and adding a pinch of salt. Cook for about 8 minutes, stirring occasionally, until the tofu begins to brown. Add mustard and dill and a tablespoon of soy sauce and cook for another 3 minutes or so, until a light crust forms on the tofu.

In another pan, heat the olive oil and sauté all the veggies for about 4 or 5 minutes, until slightly tender. Add the remaining soy sauce and tofu, stir, and cook for an additional minute or two. Serve immediately on top of the brown rice— be generous with the veggies and stingy with the rice when plating. Serves two, with leftovers for lunch the next day for one of you.

5

discipline and zeal (*tapas*)

*C'MON BABY, LIGHT YOUR (INNER) FIRE
(TAPAS: BURNING ZEAL)*

SUTRA II.I: *TAPAH SVADHYAYA
ISVARAPRANIDHANANI KRIYAYOGAH*

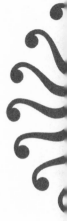

Burning zeal in practice, self-study
and study of scriptures, and
surrender to God are acts
of yoga. —B. K. S. Iyengar

Doctor Dosha

E ven when I was forty pounds overweight, I knew
somewhere deep down that I could change things
with a lot of hard work. In Nepal, during my junior year
abroad, I hadn't had a fancy trainer, special workout clothes,
access to a gym, or a carefully tailored meal plan. Just a whole
lot of walking in ratty sneaker-boots, a vegetarian diet, and a
month of fairly dramatically reducing my calorie intake and
suddenly I had—was forced by circumstances to cultivate—
an inner fire that yogis call *tapas*.

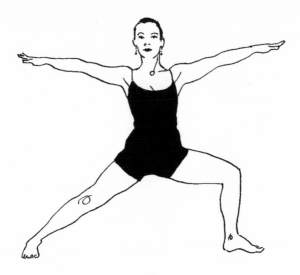

Stand with your legs about three and a half feet apart. Moving from the hip, turn your right leg until your right foot is perpendicular to your left heel. Bend your right leg until your right knee is in line with your right foot and the thigh is parallel to the floor. Keep the back left leg straight while bending the right leg closer and closer to that 90-degree angle. Make sure to have a wide-enough stance to make this possible. Raise your arms and stretch them out wide to either side, purposefully extending them as you widen and create space along your collarbones and shoulder blades. Look at the middle finger of the right hand and take steady, long breaths. Change sides and repeat with the left leg turned out. Can you take a sense of satisfaction and even pleasure in the hard work involved in this pose, even as your thighs burn?

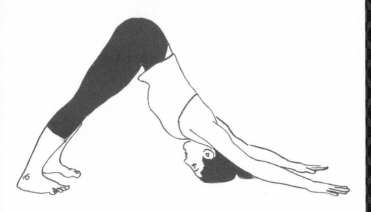

Begin on all fours. Press back onto the balls of your feet and raise your hips high as you straighten your legs. (If your hamstrings feel too tight to straighten your legs in this pose, work with bent knees.) Once in the pose, place your hands several inches wider than shoulder-distance apart, with your wrists turned slightly out. Press your palms, particularly the inside corner of each hand, firmly down and dynamically lift your weight up and out of your shoulders. Extend your hips to the ceiling and begin to straighten your legs even more. Gaze between your feet; release your neck, and breathe. Notice what it feels like to work in a focused and determined way without knowing what you look like, or having the chance to compare yourself with others.

Accepting pain as help for purification, study of spiritual books, and surrender to the Supreme Being constitutes yoga in practice.

—Sri Swami Satchidananda

One late-winter afternoon in Katmandu, after the morning frost had melted into a sunny day, my fellow students and I went on a field trip to a local doctor's office. Modest by American standards, the office contained all the basics needed for a family practice—exam table, stethoscope, stacks of gauze pads, and disinfectants. Unlike the doctors we were used to visiting at home and in our college infirmaries, however, this doctor was a practitioner of Ayurveda, the Indian science of healing. Our field trip was meant as an introduction to Eastern medicine.

The doctor explained to us that Ayurveda is a way of thinking about the body and health based on correcting imbalances and helping people find their physical and psychological equilibrium. To determine appropriate treatment for ailments, Ayurvedic practitioners start by determining the patient's constitution, or body and personality type.

There are three basic constitutions—or *doshas*—described in Ayurveda: *pittas* are fiery, hot, determined types; *vatas* are nervous and enthusiastic, lanky and quick; and *kaphas* are lethargic and earthy, solid, and comforting. Physical characteristics go along with each type. *Pittas* are generally well-proportioned, while *vatas* with their nervous energy are often on the skinny side; *kaphas*, with their peaceful and placid energy, tend to be heavier.

According to Ayurvedic doctors, most people tend toward one of these types more than the other two: Health and well-being come about when this tendency is counterbalanced by attributes from the other two types. The Nepalese physician began asking us a series of questions to determine our Ayurvedic types. As I scribbled down my answers on the questionnaire, I tried to hide them from my fellow students. I worried that since I'd had a tendency to keep extra weight on, I must be a *kapha* and was therefore *destined* to be fat, or at least fat off and on, for the rest of my life. After all, I'd had a weight problem since elementary school.

Just as I was beginning to feel *really* sorry for myself, the doctor dropped a life-changing piece of information. *Doshas are not set in stone!* The whole point of Ayurveda, he insisted, was that by changing the way we live—how we eat, move, sleep, work, and relate to others—we can balance our systems.

Austerity, study, and the dedication of the fruits of one's work to God: these are the preliminary steps towards yoga.

— Swami Prabhavananda and Christopher Isherwood

Monkey Temple

I shouldn't have needed an Ayurvedic physician to tell me that. I'd come to the Himalayas a chain-smoking, definitely-take-the-elevator kind of girl, and in just a matter of weeks my molecules seemed to be realigning. Who *was* this mountain-climbing, vegetable-and-lentil-munching, and certifiably *thin* young woman I seemed to be morphing into? It all started with a monkey temple.

During our stay in Katmandu, I was hosted by a family—a mother and father and their two young daughters—

who lived around the corner from the Swayambunath Stupa, a.k.a. the Monkey Temple. The temple was on the other side of town from the schoolhouse where we attended daily classes. A half-dozen single-gear bicycles had been made available for students like me, living on the outskirts of the city, but I was way too afraid to ride a bike through streets crammed with animals and mopeds and shop stalls and all the other things that make up the beautiful chaos of Katmandu street life. No, I decided, I'd rather walk. It might take me all day, but at least I'd avoid colliding with a cow or wandering *sadhu*, or holy man. My homestay "dad"—an architect—drew me a detailed map to show me how to get to school. I clutched the map in my hands as I walked on: left at the Monkey Temple, right at the bazaar, straight through the *dahl baht* stand and the stall selling wool sweaters to tourists. An hour and a half later I arrived at the school's courtyard and collapsed: sweaty, thirsty, and doubtful I could make the trip back home at the end of the day.

But I didn't have much choice. And, to my surprise, I came to cherish the time I spent walking. What started out as a ninety-minute walk each way soon became more like an hour as I picked up my pace and became more familiar with my route. Each day, I relaxed into the rhythms of the walk and started paying closer attention to the color-drenched, chaotic, Jessica-you're-so-not-in-Long-Island-anymore magic of Katmandu. Six weeks of walking to and from school helped me prepare for my next big challenge—a month-long independent-study period trekking in the countryside. When I signed up for the project, I didn't realize how much hiking would be involved. I began to get the picture when I set off on my travels, reading the directions my language teacher Ram had written out for me the night before: Take a twelve-hour bus ride—and then hike *for five days* (with a local guide hired on the spot) through what turned out to be, by turns, gloriously lush valleys and isolated snowy hilltops.

When I finally reached my destination, I arranged to stay with a family who had a daughter a few years younger than me. They worked as innkeepers, running a small three-room lodge in a town full of similar, mostly empty establishments. The inn was comfortable by backpacking standards—I had my own room and bed, with a bathroom out back—but there wasn't much extra food to go around. I ate what I was given for breakfast and supper, snagging some crackers from a small general store in the afternoons. I was hungry, but then so much else was strange and new for me about the experience—I didn't speak English the whole time I was in the village, and my Nepali skills were pretty basic—that the hunger seemed like just another new sensation. (Dirty? Check. In culture shock? Check. Hungry? Check. Having one of the coolest experiences of my young, sheltered life? Check.) I read the few books in my backpack over and over, wrote in my journal, went to market day in a "nearby" town that was a four- or five-hour hike away—talk about walking off lunch—and hung out at the local village holiday festival.

Cultivating *Tapas*: No Laziness Allowed

Success in yoga comes quickly to those who are intensely energetic. Success varies according to the means adopted to obtain it—mild, medium, or intense.

—Sri Swami Prabhavananda and Christopher Isherwood

Without realizing it at the time, what I was doing in Nepal was cultivating *tapas.* Swami Prabhavananda and his coauthor, artist and writer Christopher Isherwood, write in their 1953 translation of (and commentary on) the Yoga Sutras, "Buddha pointed out that, if there is any sin, it is laziness." Willpower, discipline—*tapas,* as it's called in Sanskrit—isn't a temporary way of being—it's an ongoing process, a daily choice we need to make again and again about how to live.

When it comes to eating and exercise, there's no getting around what we all know: To lose weight, you're going to have to eat much less and exercise much more. Once you're maintaining a healthy weight, eating wholesome, energy-giving foods in moderation, and integrating physical activity into your daily routine, it will all become much easier. But in the beginning, it's going to be a battle. You *will* be hungry; you *will* feel like you're spending all of your free time exercising. Everyday you'll think about giving up. That's where *tapas* comes in. Instead of feeling deprived and dejected, embrace and savor the challenge of cultivating a strong, determined, lasting inner fire.

Although yoga has always felt natural to me, I wasn't born with any particular talent for the poses and postures. My body's not especially flexible and wasn't always agile—I couldn't do a single cartwheel as a child, much less stand on my hands or head—so I had to work hard to build my yoga practice, being enthusiastic (on my best days, at least) and acquiring discipline.

Take, for example, *sirsasana*, or headstand pose. For me, no pose exhibits the beauty and grace of yoga asana more than headstand. Once I began practicing at the yoga center in New York, I made the pose my unspoken goal—even though it seemed so far away. When it came time for headstand I'd slink into a corner or take a bathroom break. One day, though, I gathered my nerve, raised a hand, and asked for my teacher's help. If I positioned myself against the wall, and my teacher lifted my legs up into the pose, I was surprised to see that I could stay up—at least for a moment.

To take the next step and make the headstand my own, however, I'd need to lift *myself* up into the air. I tried and tried in class. I even went to a special headstand workshop and spent $40 being lifted again and again. I *still* couldn't do it by myself.

Eventually, once I began studying Iyengar yoga—a precise method and style of yoga developed by yoga luminary B. K. S. Iyengar at his center in India—I learned that the key to successfully doing this intermediate posture was to work diligently on my beginning standing poses, so that I could build the strength and flexibility and sense of steadiness needed to balance in handstand. Once I did so, I learned how to gently bring my body up, stacking my torso carefully on top of my head and shoulders, lifting myself up toward the ceiling. The next step was to *stay* there. At home, I'd practice each day, staying for half a minute, and then one minute, and then two, until I could stay up for five minutes. Then, I worked on getting up and staying up without the help of the wall, just me on my own in the center of the room. It took me years to do, and I still work on turning those five minutes into ten—but today when I go up into a headstand, I know I've earned it.

Most of us have employed *tapas* in one or another area of our lives—maybe for you it's your career, or even your love life. Now you need to take this skill and apply it to the way you eat and exercise. Ask yourself: Do you really need that midnight bowl of cereal or bag of potato chips? Could you cultivate *tapas* and have an apple instead? Take the stairs instead of the elevator? Resist hopping into the car and walk? Spend the weekend snowshoeing rather than shopping? Protect that one-fourth empty feeling in your belly? Tapping into your potential for willpower and discipline is an important step on the road to becoming enlightened.

Come to know the difference between working hard at something and overdoing it. Don't hurt yourself, but don't go too easy on yourself, either.

"That's not pain," my current yoga teacher Louie Ettling likes to say. "That's a thigh stretch."

Are Your Friends Making You Fat?

Nicholas Christakis, a sociologist at Harvard, recently proved the following common-sense theory: Weight problems run in social networks. Overweight people tend to have overweight people as friends. Do people become more like those they hang out with, or are they attracted to those of a similar weight? My guess is a little of both.

Warning: Fat is Contagious

I remember how comforting it was in high school to have lunch with a close friend who'd order the same unhealthy foods as me; it made me feel less self-conscious about myself, my weight, and what I was eating. On the other hand, later in my life, when I decided to surround myself with inspiring, healthy, upbeat, and disciplined types, I was transported into my very own *Ray of Light* Madonna in the late 1990s yoga period (minus Rupert Everett and that sweet Craftsman-style cottage). Most of my friends these days eat pretty much the same way I do and don't make me feel like a health nut for suggesting a sushi lunch, or ordering fruit on the side instead of potatoes with eggs, or substituting steamed greens for toast. They're too busy ordering their egg–white–only omelets or veggie scrambles.

There's a word for this in Sanskrit: s*atsang.* On the road to enlightenment, it helps to find support. All of us would-be yogis need to hang out with like-minded people who are equally interested in health and spiritual seeking. *Satsang* is what happens during these get-togethers—the social support and solidarity that develop when yogis meet to discuss philosophy, chant, or just break out the tofu lasagna (with whole wheat noodles, of course).

Try surrounding yourself with positive, health-loving people. They don't have to be self-identified yogis; it doesn't matter if they've never cracked open a copy of the Sutras or kicked up into a handstand. Chances are you know someone at work or school or in the neighborhood who has a good attitude about exercise and a sense of restraint when it comes to food, and who, even more importantly, has her emotional life together. Follow this person around. Study her. Make her your new best friend. This isn't to say that you should shut yourself off from those in your life who aren't on the same healthy path. Unless they're truly toxic, take them under your own newly yogic wing. And don't be surprised when you find yourself being followed around town one day soon by someone inspired by—and wanting to be with—you.

Country Walks, City Walks

Instilling this new sense of discipline, this *tapas*—not just temporarily but for good—may take time. But it's a critical part of changing your lifestyle so that you can become someone who makes exercise a natural part of your daily life.

Take walking. Even after trekking in Nepal, walking everywhere was something I still had to learn to apply in my regular life back home. Like most yogic lessons, it took me a while (translation: almost an entire decade). But eventually it sunk in. Now, when it rains, I bust out my rain boots and umbrella. When it snows I wear fleece and long johns and wool sweaters under my puffy winter coat. When it's freezing, I freeze. But I keep walking. By now, my walking habit is second nature. I almost always prefer walking to driving, especially with my baby happily tucked in his baby carrier or stroller. And Salem will take a walk over a ride in the station wagon any day.

Be persistent. When a friend asks me out to coffee, I suggest a walk instead. Some of the best conversations happen during long walks, whether you're in the forest on a hiking trail or on a crowded sidewalk in the middle of the city. You don't have to live in the perfect walking town, either. Even in L.A., where driving is as much a part of life as velour tracksuits, it *is* possible to find satisfying neighborhood walks and kick-ass hikes. Neil and I have walked along the beach in Miami, in a Brooklyn park, around busy Boston streets. Traveling through India on a belated honeymoon, we walked in the early morning through Mumbai, before the heat and chaotic street life got going. If outdoor walking isn't an option because of climate or your personal weather-tolerance threshold, find your local gym or Y and get walking on the treadmill. You'll still get the cardio benefits—although you will miss out on the psychological and spiritually uplifting benefits of outdoor walking.

Baby Weight

The first steps, then, are to get moving and to stop eating so much. That said, however, depending on how much weight you have to lose, walking by itself, or even combined with yoga, might not be enough. You may need to cultivate higher-intensity *tapas*. In my case, back in the Berkshires,

I also had to put in some serious treadmill and elliptical trainer time—starting with as much as I could handle, about fifteen or twenty minutes a session, and working my way up to forty-five-minute workouts two or three times a week—in addition to walking and yoga in order to lose weight. With the forty pounds gone, I figured I'd never have to get back on the treadmill again. Walking and yoga, along with portion control and eating healthy foods, kept me thin.

Then I had a baby. When I was pregnant I kept up my yoga practice, attending prenatal classes, practicing restorative poses at home, going up into a handstand even in my last month, and taking daily hour-long walks in the park with Salem. Still, I managed to gain more than forty-five pounds. Let's just say that when it came to my pregnancy, I was channeling Kate Hudson, not Nicole Kidman.

In the first half of my pregnancy, all I could stomach was food I'd previously put the kibosh on: bagels, potato chips, milkshakes, heaping bowls of light-as-air Cheerios, which I hadn't had since our early-couplehood days of "snack." My body seemed determined to build up fat reserves. One week early in my first trimester I gained ten—yes, ten!—pounds, going from 112 to 122 in seven days. That's a whole lot of Cheerios. I'd try to eat my super-healthy staples, but I'd throw up before the meal was half done. My been-there-done-that, skinny-again mommy friends told me not to worry and offered me an array of what I hoped weren't just excuses: I had fertility drugs in my system; I was thin to start out with and needed to gain more than the average amount of weight. They promised me that I'd return to normal a few months after giving birth.

Besides, after trying for years to have a baby, wasn't it beyond petty to care about something as superficial as weight gain and the size of my maternity jeans?

Right or wrong, I *did* care. I knew what it felt like to be overweight, and I didn't want to go down that road again. And, as important as it is to eat enough when pregnant and not worry about gaining a normal amount of weight— twenty-five to forty pounds for women of average weight, more if you're underweight, and less if you're overweight before becoming pregnant—it's equally important not to gain *too* much weight. Recent research by Dr. Teresa A. Hillier, an endocrinologist at the Kaiser Permanente Center for Health Research in Portland, Oregon, shows that women who gain too much weight during pregnancy have larger babies, who themselves become more likely to be overweight or obese as children and adults.

Even my obstetrician mentioned that I might want to keep an eye on the scale. "How about only eating *half* a bagel for breakfast?" she bargained. I wanted a child more than anything, but I also hoped to be a healthy, active mom. Certainly, I didn't want to pass on to my child the obesity that was common in my family. So, after a few months, once the morning sickness had abated, I limited my empty-calorie treats and tried to pack wholesome calories into my meals and snacks—no more bagels and milkshakes except on the rare occasion, more veggies and fruits, and lots of whole grains and protein (salmon, tofu, legumes). The nausea returned during the last couple weeks of my pregnancy, and I regressed. All I could hold down was chocolate frozen yogurt, elbow macaroni with plain tomato sauce (hello, childhood!), and my old friends, those lightly toasted sesame bagels swabbed with cream cheese.

I stopped getting on the scale.

When I did weigh myself, a week or so postpartum (I know, I know, I shouldn't have!), I did a double take. To get back down to my pre-pregnancy weight, I'd have to lose thirty pounds. I'd heard that baby weight was the easiest kind of weight to lose, but *thirty pounds*? I couldn't even pull on the absurdly overpriced designer maternity jeans I'd splurged on after my twelve-week sonogram in a fit of maternal insanity.

But baby weight wasn't the main problem. Like many a yoga-loving mom-to-be before me, I'd imagined a drug-free, midwife-attended birth in which I'd gracefully breathe and position and visualize myself through the contractions until I eased my baby out into the world, perhaps in a bath-tub. Instead, I ended up with a long and difficult labor and an unplanned C-section. Afterward, because I'd had a fever and a long labor and had needed IV antibiotics, Lucien was whisked away to the NICU for forty-eight hours. I had to get my drugged-out, aching, and sore self down there every two hours if I wanted any chance at nursing him.

We went home from the hospital as soon as they released him, only to find that my legs had swollen to three times their normal size. No exaggeration: Neil could no longer distinguish my knees from the rest of my legs. So Neil, Lucien, and I spent the first night "home" camped out in the emergency room of the very same hospital I'd checked out of mere hours before. While we waited to see a doctor, me nursing in a bathroom, I broke down.

"I've waited so long to have this baby, and he's here and he's perfect, and all I want is to be his mother, and now I'm going to die!"

It must have been the Percocet talking.

Later that morning we went to see my obstetrician, who assured me that even elephantine swelling was within the bounds of normal after a C-section, especially an unplanned one that came after a long labor. I was grateful to be okay and overjoyed to head home with Lucien, but I was also feeling physically wrecked by the combination of IVF, the pregnancy, and the birth. How would I take care of my baby?

Much more important than fitting into a pair of jeans, I told myself, was to figure out how to once again feel healthy and strong. Geeta Iyengar, the modern day guru of Iyengar yoga for women, and daughter of B. K. S. Iyengar, advises new mothers who are recovering from a C-section to practice only the most restful and healing restorative poses in the six months after surgery. (Moms need to take it easy after vaginal births, too, although they can start their yoga practice— slowly and carefully—after six weeks.)

But I couldn't see how I'd be practicing yoga again in six years, much less six months. My torso was numb; I couldn't feel much of anything between my breasts and my hips besides my sore and aching scar. Getting out of bed and carrying my baby over to the changing table was difficult for me, and the walk to our pediatrician's office several blocks away took more willpower than some of my treks through Nepal. To be the healthy and strong mom I wanted to be, and to eventually practice yoga again, I'd need to not only lose the baby weight but also strengthen my core and build my abdominals back.

Easier said than done.

Complicating matters, *I was still hungry!* There was no way I was going to starve myself and potentially mess with my milk supply. Lucien was slow to gain weight, and we were taking him to twice-weekly weigh-ins. I had to have a lactation consultant come over and help me with nursing techniques. The challenge for me, as for most new moms, was to balance the need to lose weight and get back in shape with the need to keep my calories and energy up for breast-feeding. For me, this meant a careful but calorie-generous nutritional plan, and some serious exercise. If I ever needed *tapas*, this would be the time.

But my body felt foreign, weak, and strange.

My friend Katherine, who'd been through three C-sections herself, told me I *had* to get out of bed, off the painkillers, and start walking. "I promise you, Jess," Kathy said, "that's the only way to get strong again." We'd been friends since the seventh grade, and she'd never given me bad advice, so I decided to trust her.

One weekend, at five weeks postpartum, I attempted a three-mile walk around the park with the stroller. This was huge; before this, I'd hardly made it down the block. I packed enough baby supplies for a day out with quintuplets: two changes of clothes, diapers of the cloth, chlorine free, *and* Disney-cartoon-adorned varieties; nursing blanket, spit-up cloth, fleece bunting, water bottle for Mommy, windbreaking stroller cover. I dragged Neil along, too, just in case I couldn't finish the loop all the way around and needed help getting the stroller into a taxi. Sweat dripped down me as I walked, soaking through the two pairs of sports bras I'd rigged together in an attempt to support my new size-D breasts. I moaned and complained to Neil every other minute that I'd never make it.

And then, just when I was about to demand that Neil call the paramedics, we turned a corner and there it was— the end of the loop. Hare Krishna! I was sore and thirsty

and my sweatshirt was drenched with sweat, but the fire re-
newed inside me felt so good. After that, Lucien and I hit
the park on our own most days, rounding the loop in shorter
and shorter times, stopping only for nursing breaks and dia-
per changes on some cold park benches. Each walk was easier than the one before. Salem, as you can imagine, happily
tagged along. I juggled the leash, the stroller, and recyclable
poop bags all while listening to my cheesy hit-the-park mix
of Kelly, Kanye, and Justin. On good days, I even managed
to stop worrying about my scar.

Although the walks were a great first step, I had a nag-
ging suspicion that I needed more than just walking. At seven
weeks postpartum I took my first Mommy-and-Baby exercise class at a small neighborhood gym a few blocks from us.
(I'd put myself on the list for class before giving birth, which
was a good thing, as I can't imagine having had the time
or energy to figure out where to go after bringing Lucien
home.) I struggled and sweated through every minute and
literally cried on the way home from exhaustion and frustra-
tion. A single sit-up was completely beyond me. The surgery
had left my entire midsection numb. I couldn't even *feel* my
core, belly, or abs post–C-section, much less engage them.

Mommy-and-baby fitness classes weren't necessarily
how I wanted to spend three mornings a week, especially
after being up most of the night with the baby. What I really
craved—and what the *kapha* in me felt I *deserved*—was to

put the baby in a sling and head to the local bakery, where I could drink coffee and snack on bagels with the other mommies. But, lovely as a morning baked good sounded, not only was the exercise helping me to get back in shape, it was also helping me adapt to the physiological challenges of new motherhood, keeping my mood and energy up. Because of my history of depression, Neil and I were worried I'd have postpartum problems. But thanks to all the endorphins from exercise, combined with the oxytocin from nursing, I was feeling surprisingly great (for someone who'd had major abdominal surgery several weeks earlier).

Not wanting to mess with success, I got used to plunking Lucien down on the gym floor with the babies of other health-nutty mommies. He'd look at me quizzically as I did my cardio drills and squat thrusts. A couple of days a week, I hit the treadmill and jogged, handing Lucien off to a burly guy named Mo who worked the front desk.

Thankfully, though not surprisingly, healthy eating plus a lot of exercise = weight loss. Before long, the designer maternity jeans came on; within another six weeks, they were too loose on me. I was glad to be making my way down the scale again, but I still had a good fifteen or twenty pounds to go. I decided to give myself three months of serious *tapas* extra credit assignments: I signed up for a dozen personal training sessions (my "push" present, something that we budgeted for in advance); kept a food diary, eating lots of wild salmon and greens and lentils, and dropping bread products entirely; walked Lucien around the park about a zillion times; and, embarrassingly enough, watched *The Biggest Loser* for inspiration while nursing at three in the morning.

By Lucien's six-month birthday I'd lost almost all the baby weight, aside from the five or so pounds my baby books said my body might want to keep in reserve for breastfeeding. By ten months postpartum, most of those pounds came off me, too, without much special effort. Of course, my body's different than it was before. Some of my skinniest "skinny" jeans are a bit too snug in the tummy and behind; my body, overall, is more rounded, a bit less hard and flat. Some of my pre-pregnancy clothes fit, and some don't—and you know what? I don't mind.

I'm able to carry around my growing child, I'm back to my five-minute headstands, and I'm feeling healthy and strong again. After I lost the baby weight, I said good-bye to the gym and returned to my daily regimen of walking and yoga.

Find Your Yoga

While yoga, in combination with walking or other cardiovascular movement, is incredibly effective for maintaining your weight and staying healthy, the wisdom behind the physical practice can help you as much as the poses can—maybe more. You don't need to do a downward dog every day to balance your *dosha*, or find your inner fire. Maybe what you need is a kickboxing session or to take a dance class one or two nights a week. Just like everyone needs her own version of veggie chili, the staple food that keeps your digestive system healthy and fueled, we each need to find our own yoga, the physical work that keeps us healthy and strong.

Bun Head

Back in college I did have one friend who somehow knew—even as a teenager—not just how to be disciplined but how to channel her discipline and *tapas* in a positive direction. Compared to me, it was like she came from a different planet. Jenna was my token "healthy" friend. While the rest of my friends and I drank tall forties of cheap beer and smoked a pack of cigarettes a day, Jenna went to bed early and woke up a few hours after the rest of us stumbled home. On top of her course load, she had to be up early for a rigorous schedule of dance rehearsals; she was a member of the college's modern dance company. When she had the rare day free, she did seemingly odd things like hiking. I enjoyed hanging out with Jenna, but I didn't make any serious attempts to emulate her healthy lifestyle. There was no way I could ever be like her, I figured, so why try? Me: depressed, black-clad, bad-poetry-writing, more often than not overweight. Jenna: avocado-and-apple-eating health nut with the ability to fly across a stage.

Years later, we reconnected. Now that I was getting healthy and disciplined myself, Jenna no longer seemed so exotic. All of the sudden she was someone I could relate to more than my other college friends, many of whom continued the hard-living habits we'd honed at school.

As we caught up on each other's news, I learned that Jenna had gone through her own struggles. Too often, women can go overboard once they become disciplined and veer into body-image problems and even eating disorders. For Jenna, these issues came up in the world of ballet, which she'd entered as a young girl. She loved to dance; she loved the process of learning and integrating choreography, the way the movements felt in her body. But as she grew older and started to develop hips and thighs and breasts, the pressure to look a certain undersized way kicked in. And by older, I'm not talking about eighteen or nineteen. In Jenna's high-intensity New Jersey dance school, the teachers encouraged *nine-year-olds* to stay super-skinny.

Things got worse as she grew older. When Jenna was eleven, her teacher, a former prima ballerina, poked Jenna's tummy and behind with a dance stick and told her she could tell she'd eaten spaghetti for dinner the previous day. Later that year Jenna asked her teacher why she was always picked for the boy rather than the girl roles; her teacher said it was because her legs were too "thick and bulky" for the girls' parts and that she "wouldn't look right in a tutu." Two years later, at age thirteen, Jenna got sick and lost a lot of weight over the course of a long winter. The ballet company rewarded her with her first tutu role.

She got the message.

Eventually Jenna regained those few pounds, returning to a healthy weight. At the age of fourteen she took a look at her body—her strong thighs and relatively short (when compared to an impossibly tall ballerina type) legs—and decided that she wasn't willing to sacrifice her self-esteem and self-worth to ballet. Instead of coveting a ballerina's body, or career, she'd make her own path—one where she could dance, live at a sensible weight, and enjoy her body's abilities and grace rather than hate herself for not being born with a "proper" ballet silhouette. She cut off her ballet bun and started wearing her hair short, packed up her pointe shoes, and made the switch to modern dance—where her so-called thick legs were suddenly an asset, a sign of strength and beauty. She danced in the company at Vassar and then, after college, in San Francisco.

Now thirty-five, Jenna's a mom and a pilates teacher living in Pasadena, California. Jenna credits her own mother's healthy habits as the main reason she didn't get sucked into a heavy-duty psychological complex around body issues, or an eating disorder. She recently shared with me in an e-mail that her mom "is extremely healthy and balanced in her eating and exercising. She made all our breads, cookies, and dinners from scratch using ingredients from the hippie food co-op that she was a member of. She even ground her own grain for a while! She started exercising right at the beginning of the exercise boom, taking aerobics classes like Jane Fonda in thong leotards. I never once heard her complain about her body. She always told me I was strong and beautiful. She never commented on anyone else's weight. And that I basically idolized her—even through my teen years—made me take after her in many ways."

Now, not all of us are going to grow up with parents who have the time or the inclination to grind their own grain, but we *can* follow Jenna's example in smaller ways. For starters, try not allowing the culture around you to dictate your unhealthy food habits or create for you an unrealistic body image. Instead of focusing on being stick-skinny, endeavor to be strong, healthy, and to feel alive and happy in your body.

Jenna doesn't have many food hang-ups, and neither should you! You can eat bread—*once in a while.* Of course, good food should be enjoyed. Make whole wheat bread a special treat. The homemade kind, made with care and love in your kitchen, can be especially satisfying. Here's a recipe from Jenna's mom, something she made for Jenna when she was a child. Enjoy each bite, in moderation.

Honey Wheat Bread, recipe and tips from Jenna's mom, a.k.a. Louise Marshall

Makes two loaves.

3 cups wheat flour *

1/2 cup dry nonfat milk powder

1 tablespoon salt

2 packages of yeast **

3 cups water***

1/2 cup honey (a light-colored, mild-flavored honey is best)

2 tablespoons oil (same for the oil; canola is good, as is safflower; use expeller-pressed, preferably organic)

4 to 4 1/2 cups all-purpose white flour

Combine first four ingredients in large mixer bowl. Heat water, honey, and oil in a pan until very warm, but not hot (you should be able to stick your finger in it and keep it there for a couple of seconds).

With a handheld mixer, blend at low speed for 1 minute, and medium speed for 2 minutes. By hand, gradually stir in 1 additional cup of wheat flour and 4 to 4 1/2 cups all-purpose white flour. Turn out onto floured board and knead until smooth and glossy, but not sticky.

Place in greased bowl. Cover with a folded towel (not touching the dough) and let rise in a warm place for 45 to 60 minutes. You'll know the dough has risen enough if, when you poke a hole in it with your finger, the hole remains in the dough.

Shape into two loaves by dividing equally in half, rolling out each half into a large rectangle (one dimension must be the length of your bread pan), and then tightly rolling up the rectangle. Place seam side down into two greased full-size bread pans. Let rise 30 to 45 minutes. If you desire, the pans can be loosely covered with plastic wrap and placed in the refrigerator for up to 12 hours until you are ready to bake.

Bake in preheated 375-degree oven for 40 to 45 minutes. Tent with foil if the tops are getting too dark. Bread is done when it sounds hollow when you tap it. Turn out onto racks to cool. Eat and enjoy!

* Buy the freshest bread flour (made from spring wheat) you can find. The best is to buy your own wheat berries and grind them yourself. Second best is from a store with a large turnover. There is no third best.

** For a cool-rise (refrigerator-rise) method, the best yeast to use is active dry yeast or starter yeast (i.e., a sourdough or sponge). Do not use instant yeast or rapid-rise yeast for the cool-rise method.

*** Here's another nutritional hint: When cooking certain vegetables for your family (these would include peas, corn, potatoes, and carrots—not broccoli, spinach, or strong-flavored vegetables, however), save the water (because it has all the vitamins) and freeze it. When you're ready to make bread, thaw that veggie water and use it in the bread. They will never know! And the sugars in that water will give you a higher and lighter loaf. Whatever you do, don't use strongly flavored veggie water, such as broccoli, spinach, etc. If you don't use veggie water, be sure to use pure filtered water.

Professor of Yoga

There are so many ways to move like a yogi. Like Jenna, you can dance and hike and practice pilates. On the other hand, I can't say enough about the benefits and joys of the actual practice of yoga. Yoga has profoundly changed my life, and the lives of many of my friends and acquaintances.

Yoga poses have an amazing ability to open up your body, your heart, and your mind—even for the most cerebral among us.

Neil's friend Mitchell is a sociologist with a five-times-a-week-yoga-class habit. He didn't start practicing yoga until his late thirties, but it's made a huge difference in his life. As a boy, Mitchell was more than a little self-conscious about himself and his body. For one thing, he was overweight. For another, he was gay at a time when that still carried with it a crushing load of social stigma.

As a teenager Mitchell was determined to thin down. He started running. For years, he ran and ran hard—three miles one day, eight miles another; he'd hit the track or trail four or five days a week. Not only did he get thin, but the running also provided a focus to his day, and a mental clarity that helped him succeed well into graduate school. But by the time he moved to New York City at age thirty-six to take a job at New York University, he faced a turning point when it came to both his home life and his body. He was going through a break up and had a growing sense that his knees were not going to let him run this hard for another twenty years.

Anxious and depressed, Mitchell tried everything—re-uptake inhibitors, swimming, therapy, daily visits to the gym. Medication and therapy helped, but swimming and working out never gave him the anxiety-reducing benefits he'd found through running. He experimented with yoga off and on, and then three years ago found a yoga center that made the practice click for him. Mitchell started going to class more and more regularly.

Since getting his yoga on, Mitchell tells me he's become calmer and more focused than at any other time in his life. His body looks and feels better than ever, too. "It's been a mental and physical transformation," Mitchell says, "but a gradual, unplanned one." These days he's much less interested in fancy foods and is happiest with simple, small, and more-frequent meals. A former hard-core cigarette smoker, he's down to just the very occasional cigarette, too. For Mitchell, as for me (and so many others whose lives have been transformed by something as ostensibly simple as a series of stretches), yoga is a prescription for staying healthy and balanced. It's physically calming, mentally contemplative and recharging, and "the secret to aging gracefully," according to Mitchell. As he puts it, yoga is "fundamentally simple—endlessly complex—and intellectually stimulating." Now if only he could convince Neil to attend class more regularly . . .

Whether you decide to make a habit of yoga asana practice or not, cultivating *tapas* is an essential step toward losing weight and getting healthy.

Getting Started: Tips for Balancing that *Dosha* and Lighting Your Inner Fire

- **Think Thin, or WWYD?**

Think like the healthy, disciplined person you are in the process of becoming. Ask yourself, before ordering food, or deciding whether or not to exercise, *What Would a Yogi Do?*

- **Start Moving Every Day**

When working to lose weight, exercise three to five times a week; make sure to break a sweat and work to your maximum. Your clothes should be damp after a hard-core workout. Take an exercise class; run on the treadmill; do the elliptical machine; play soccer or basketball; jog in your neighborhood. Walk everywhere. Begin a yoga practice—at home, with the poses suggested in this book, as well as a class with a good, experienced teacher.

- **Hit the Road**

No matter where you live, and whether you're trying to lose or simply maintain your weight, start walking. No excuses. You don't need special shoes—although a pair of sneakers are nice, as is a warm coat in the winter and a good supportive bra for those who need one. You also don't need as much spare time as you'd think. Wake up an hour or even a half-hour earlier and take a meditative morning stroll. Speed-walk to work. Walk your kids to school. Walk to the playground. Walk to the gym to go run on the treadmill. For extra credit and karma points, walk to yoga class!

- **Substitute a Smoothie**

When you're heading to a workout, or just back from one, you may be better off with a mini-meal than something more substantial that could weigh you down. Smoothies make a great morning or mid-afternoon snack, or even a light lunch when paired with a protein/carbohydrate snack like a brown rice cake with almond butter. (But a word of caution: Don't think of a smoothie as a beverage to go along with your regular meal; it's substantial enough to stand on its own.) According to the trainers who helped me get my baby weight off, it's important to have something nutritious to eat two hours before exercising—any closer and you may end up with stomach cramps—and within a half-hour after a serious cardio or strength-training session, like a yoga class or vigorous walk or jog.

- **Run Off-Leash**

You don't *need* a dog to get enlightened—but it doesn't hurt. Grab your dog (or borrow a friend's) and take her to a park or yard or trail where she—and you—can run off-leash. Grab a ball or a stick and bring out your inner seven-year-old with a high-energy game of chase and fetch. You'll get some cardio and make the animal in your life healthy and happy, too. Or take your dog on a hike or a jog and turn her into your very own personal trainer.

Jessica's Midday Smoothie

One banana

1/2 cup low-fat or nonfat organic plain yogurt

1 cup frozen organic strawberries (or other available fruit)

1/4 cup organic orange juice

Honey to taste

Place ingredients in blender, mix, and enjoy!

6

purity, cleanliness (*sauca*)

ORGANIC OFFERINGS (OR, IF YOUR BODY IS A
TEMPLE, WOULD YOU REALLY WANT TO LEAVE
DORITOS AT THE ALTAR?)
(SAUCA: PURITY, CLEANLINESS)

SUTRA II.40: SAUCAT SVANGAJUGUPSA
PARAIH ASAMSARGAH

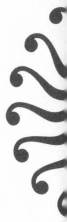

When cleanliness is developed it reveals what needs to be constantly maintained and what is eternally clean. What decays is the external. What does not is deep within us. Our over-concern with and attachment to outward things, which is both transient and superficial, is reduced. —T. K. V. Desikachar

The Kripalu Yoga Center in Lenox, Massachusetts, sits on a hill overlooking trees and a lake—a classic postcard scene with changing leaves in autumn, snowy white winters, and humid, sun-soaked summer days. When we lived in the Berkshires, I'd drive by the center on my way to teach yoga class at the ritzier, though more antiseptic, Canyon Ranch and daydream about attending my first

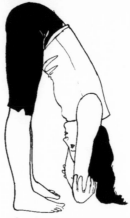

Stand with your feet firmly planted, as in mountain pose. Lift your arms up overhead, keeping them parallel and shoulder-width apart. Roll your shoulders down into the back, bringing the flesh and muscles of the upper back closer into the bone. Take hold of your elbows with opposite hands on opposite elbows. Keeping your legs active, pull up through the kneecaps and through the tops of your thighs; fold over at the hips into a standing forward bend. Tune into the give-and-take between your strong, straight legs, and the release of the forward bend—it's the stability of your foundation that provides the room and space for that sense of freedom and release. For a deeper sense of relaxation, try a supported version of this same pose by resting the top of your head on a yoga block, stack of books, or on a chair, and remain here for three to five minutes. Either way, as you allow the benefits of this inversion to wring the impurities out of your system, enjoy the yoga high—free, always good, and, unlike my old marijuana habit, highly legal.

Kripalu retreat. Just the thought of Kripalu was (and is) enough to lower my blood pressure by ten points and leave me with the urge to give away my worldly possessions and spend my days wearing comfy yoga pants and Indian blouses and sipping tea while having calm, quiet conversations about spiritual uplift.

When a new Kripalu catalog would come in the mail, I'd paw the glossy pages, an eager if cash-poor supplicant. One chilly spring before we had Lucien, I decided to go for it, bunking in the communal dorm-like rooms to save money. Hoping to find more clarity regarding my relationship to food, I signed up for an old-school Kripalu juice fast.

Saucha is inner and outer cleanliness of the body. . . . Eating simple and nutritious foods rather than food which titillates the palate is . . . a simple factor of external purity without which inner cleanliness or cleanliness of the mind cannot be achieved.

—Geeta Iyengar

The Fruits of Fasting

Reading up on Ayurveda, I learned that a juice fast would be a safe and healthy way for me to explore the psychological aspects of my food and weight issues. Dr. Vasant Lad—an Ayurvedic physician and director of the Ayurvedic Institute in Albuquerque, New Mexico—told me more when I called him for an article I was writing. Dr. Lad explained that unhealthy, unbalanced diets are often the result of mental toxins, or *ama*. To re-create balance in the body and mind, he recommended burning *ama* by fasting—known in Ayurveda as *kshut nigraha* (holding or controlling one's hunger). But physicians of Ayurveda, including Dr. Lad and his colleague, Dr. Robert Svoboda (author of a great book on Ayurveda for women), warn that even though fasting can be beneficial, for most people it shouldn't be taken to extremes. A water-only fast, for example, could shock and deplete the system rather than replenish it. A fruit and/or vegetable juice fast is a more stable method of cleansing.

I wasn't sure what to expect when I arrived at Kripalu, but I didn't have to wait long before my eating habits were turned upside down. The first morning of the program we spent more than thirty minutes drinking a single glass of juice. Alison Shore Gaines, a senior faculty member and director of the fast, was leading us through an exercise in conscious sipping.

To consciously eat or drink, she said, is to bring sacredness to the act of eating by approaching each mouthful with gratitude, carefully observing how mind and body respond to the nourishment. Following Alison's instructions, my classmates and I put our glasses down in between sips, taking time to make drinking juice a meditation. Alison told us that we should practice this new consciousness with each small portion of broth, juice, and grains we would receive during the week.

It was unnerving to drink so slowly. After all, I was used to downing a juice while talking on the phone or blow-drying my hair or driving my car or checking my e-mail. Plus, I was already hungry and it was only the first morning. "What do you want out of the next sip?" Alison asked. I wanted to be comforted, I wanted to be filled. (To be honest, I wanted a grilled cheese sandwich.)

I'm not going to lie. At first, the juice fast sucked. We were given a cup of plain, bland potassium broth in the mornings, evenings, and at the time of day formerly known as lunch. Once in the late morning, and once in the early afternoon, two glasses of freshly juiced fruits or vegetables would arrive. Small portions of whole grains—brown rice or quinoa—were offered three times a day, and it was suggested that those of us who were new to fasting or in need of the grounding or stabilization that grains provide take them. That would be me. Every time they were offered, I spooned a small handful into my bowl, slowly chewing until it became liquid. Some of the others stuck to the juice and broth.

Ayurveda teaches that when fasting begins, toxins are released. I quickly learned how tangible an experience burning through *ama* can be. Even with the grains, my body crashed into detox mode. I had many of the classic signs we were warned about in the orientation session—fatigue, chills, short-lived but piercing headaches, sensitivity to noise, people, and almost all outside stimulation. The remedy, according to Alison and juice fast codirector Atma Jo Ann Levitt, RN (and author of *The Kripalu Cookbook*, a good source for healthy recipes), was to give myself an enema. Every day.

In *panchakarma*, an Ayurvedic technique for purifying the system, enemas are often used to remove toxins from the body—flushing the bowels and clearing away stagnant debris (what Alison called "toxic sludge"). Alison and Atma had us work with a basic warm-water enema, assuring us that it would do the job of moving the *ama* through. Personally, I was more concerned about my ability to get the job done, as the enemas were to be self-administered. Once I figured out the mechanics of the procedure, the enema turned out to be a less-formidable obstacle than I'd imagined, though I never exactly looked forward to my time on the bathroom floor. I tried to make it as nurturing an experience as possible, though. After the enema was done I'd take a hot shower, put on fresh clothes, and nap, read, or meditate before our next juice or broth or group meeting.

During the first few days of the fast I kept up a full activity schedule, participating in a morning walk and yoga and movement class, even though I felt weak and exhausted. By the third day, I realized that pushing myself was not the answer. I needed to relax, give myself a break from the endless cycle of doing.

Though I did feel tired, to my surprise I wasn't all that hungry. My belly didn't burn in the way I had imagined it might. Instead, strangely, I felt nourished, fed by a kind look or warm talk with a fellow faster, nurtured by a massage or a trip to the sauna, comforted by turning in early for the extra rest my body craved.

Come morning, I'd wrap myself in layers of long underwear, sweaters, and sweats and make my way to the Kripalu chapel, where our group met for workshops on topics like healing, nutrition, and asana. By day four I was bone-weary, so I was happy to see that we were scheduled to spend the morning in a conscious breathing exercise. *Ah, a light morning*, I thought to myself. It turned out to be anything but.

Alison and Atma instructed us to stretch out on the floor with blankets and pillows, and they told us that program assistants would be circulating around the room in case we needed help during the exercise. Help? What kind of help would we need? Lying on the floor was something I could handle on my own. But as we began to relax deeply, taking in deep diaphragmatic breaths—each one bigger than the last—all sorts of locked-up feelings and memories started to come up for everyone. Fits of giggles swept the room for a time. Then the mood changed. Nervous laughter turned to sobs as old traumas were revisited.

I was uncomfortable from the start. The one woman in the group I'd been trying to avoid all week had set up shop with her blankets and pillows next to me. Something about her hit home, reminding me of the part of myself I tried hardest to avoid. And here she was next to me, crying like the others. I couldn't breathe; my deliciously peaceful week of introspection and lightness was shattered by her sobs.

"I've been a bad mother . . . I'm sorry. I'm so, so sorry," she cried. It was then I realized why I'd been avoiding her. She reminded me of my own mother.

It had been liberating to leave my father behind, but it was more difficult to walk away from my mother, her pain and guilt so ripe I could taste it on my tongue. And next to me, here on the chapel floor, was a woman who reminded me of her, begging for forgiveness. I desperately wanted to leave the room, but I felt trapped. Not knowing what to do, I reached for Atma as she walked by my spot on the floor. She came to sit by me, cupping my head in her hands, soothing me, telling me that I was safe. She stayed with me as I started to sob, mothering me in a way, though she was a stranger. When it was all over she gave me a big hug. "You'll see," she told me. "This will be huge for you—a breakthrough."

And it was. As we got up to leave the chapel, I felt an incredible sense of release. Dr. Lad writes that "if a person has deep-seated, unresolved anger, fear, anxiety, grief, or sadness, these also affect the internal organs and create bodily imbalances." All along, but especially right after I broke from my parents, I'd been eating to comfort myself, to protect myself, to cover up my anger and relieve my hurt and sadness. What I realized in that moment on the carpeted chapel floor was that I could be comforted in a profound way *without food*. There I was, moving from pretty extreme emotional distress to a space of calm and peace without the intervention of pizza or french fries. Atma's soothing words and touch had been important, but what had really done it for me was regaining a sense of connection with what it is we all share—greater consciousness—or what the Sutras call the *purusha*, divine self. Cleansing myself, I'd peeled back a layer of hurt and come closer to a core of love.

Pulling myself together after the morning's exercise, I left the chapel, took a sauna, bathed, and changed into a black bodysuit and a new silk robe of pinks and purples, a gift from Neil. I felt clean and shiny and beautiful. Fellow fasters, seeing me walk through the center as if in a ball of light, asked what had happened. I couldn't put it into words until later that afternoon when I went to Kripalu's healing arts center for a foot massage.

"How do you feel?" the massage therapist asked.

"Like I'm on a magic carpet ride," I said. And I was. I was floating, flying, blissing out on lightness.

I had planned to stay on at Kripalu after the fast for a weekend yoga workshop. I worried, though, about being too exhausted from the fast to practice. To my surprise, once back on my mat I felt liquid and happy and more flexible than ever. My asana practice never felt so good.

I know what you're thinking: You don't have the money or time to attend a seven-day fast or even a weekend yoga retreat. Now, as a new mom with writing deadlines, teaching responsibilities, and bills to pay, I don't either. But there *are* ways—inexpensive, more or less simple ways—we can all start to clean up our diets, and in so doing, come to rethink our relationship with food.

Dahl Baht

Back in Nepal, dinner just about every night was *dahl baht*. Out of steaming vats and huge covered pots emerged a warm whole wheat tortilla called *chapatti* alongside heaps of cooked cauliflower and potatoes, with a spicy sauce of tomato and chili peppers, a darker, grainier rice than I was used to, and warming, fragrant lentil soup called *dahl*, which we were instructed to pour on top of everything else on our tray. We ate with clean hands (no utensils), instead using the thinly rolled *chapatti* to scoop up all the vegetables.

It was incredible, delicious—the best meal I'd ever had. In the coming months I'd devour variation after variation of this perfect (and spicy) meal—vegetables, rice, lentils, spices—once or twice a day. In Nepal, *dahl baht* is usually eaten in the late morning and then again around dinnertime. If you needed one, you'd have a modest snack at midday, like a one-egg veggie scramble with some milk tea.

One of the many fantastic things about *dahl baht* was that I could eat *a lot* of it—my host families wouldn't take no for an answer when it came to seconds—and still lose weight. When you're eating delicious, low-fat, high-fiber food, and getting plenty of exercise, you don't have to worry so much about counting calories.

A high-fiber diet, according to Marion Nestle, promotes the body's ability to digest and metabolize glucose. As Nestle explains in *What to Eat*, eating too many refined starches and sugars causes the pancreas to overproduce insulin. "As a result blood sugar drops too far (making you feel hungry). Also, muscle cells start resisting taking in more glucose, and this means more of this sugar is stored as fat. The result is that you put yourself at risk for weight gain, diabetes (the adult, type 2 variety), cardiovascular disease, and other such problems. Fiber slows down the absorption of glucose from the small intestine, which is why a diet high in fiber-containing fruits, vegetables, and grains helps keep such health problems at bay."

When I asked her to elaborate, Nestle explained that lentils like *dahl*, or the black beans in my veggie chili, contain some unusable calories in the form of indigestible fibers. That's why these foods fill you up while also promoting weight loss.

Lesson from Nepal

Whether it's *dahl baht* or veggie chili or a stir-fry straight from the bins at the farmers' market—what matters most is the overarching lesson I learned from a semester's eating in Nepal: Fill up on vegetables prepared in a healthy, low-fat way; include good fats in moderation; use spices rather than saturated fats for extra flavor, whole grains for stability and grounding, and lentils for protein. You don't have to go on a juice fast to eat clean and purify your insides.

A corollary principle to the *dahl baht* lesson is this: If you eat healthy and low-fat *most* of the time, you can splurge on the occasional more-indulgent foods. Remember, the yogi strives for moderation. And that means that once in a while you can and *should* stray from your regularly scheduled program. On a weekend—not every weekend, but on the occasional Sunday—Neil and I will go out for whole wheat organic pizza made with hormone-free cheese (I know, I live on the edge). Because I eat super-healthy the rest of the time, I know I can go for it and not gain weight. My other favorite splurges include salmon fish tacos from a shack on the pier; vegan village feast night at our favorite Indian restaurant; wild tuna on a multigrain baguette; a really good veggie burger; and a cup of hot chocolate with skim milk.

Peace, Love, and Pineapples

My all-time favorite food, though, as I've said already, is pineapple. Fruit is the ultimate cleansing and purifying food; eating it feels like giving your digestive tract a spa treatment. The fiber cleans you out and the bulk of the fruit fills you up.

While fruits (including pineapple) do contain sugars, as Michael Pollan explains in his book *In Defense of Food*, "In the natural world, fructose [sugar] . . . comes packaged in a whole food full of fiber (which slows its absorption) and valuable micronutrients." Meaning, there's a world of difference between the sugar in candy bars or your sugar jar and the sugar in an apple or pineapple. Your body can handle whole fruit sugars, at least in common-sense moderation (although you should avoid fruit juice which has too much sugar and too little fiber compared to an actual piece of fruit). These days, our household can go through three or four pineapples a week. (Everyone but Salem loves them.)

There's something so satisfying, even steak-like (tofu steak, that is), about pineapple.

Nowadays I'll often begin my morning with steel-cut oatmeal mixed with a half tablespoon of honey, some raisins for iron, and half a banana, and then have my pineapple bowl later on in the mid-morning. Occasionally, I'll even have a second big bowl of fresh fruit and yogurt for lunch, particularly in summer when my usual lunch of a lentil soup or veggie stir-fry leftovers seems too heavy, or if I'm rushed for time. Eating small meals every few hours, particularly in the morning, is a great way to keep your energy up and keep from overdoing it later on in the day—something that happens to me even now if I don't take the time and effort to eat enough early in the day. (I used to have the problem of eating too much, but with a young baby and busy schedule, simply finding the time to eat has become a new challenge. Skipping meals can lead to serious overeating come nighttime, so a filling and healthy breakfast and a mid-morning meal, as nutritionists suggest, really is essential.)

Now, eating half a pineapple a day can get pricey. But it's worth it to me to feel energetic and ready to go every morning, and the truth is that two or three bucks for a serving, plus the cost of a couple spoonfuls of yogurt and almonds, is still cheaper than buying a sandwich or breakfast out somewhere. And I save money by not needing to trade my clothes in every other year as I yo-yo up and down the scale.

Tips for Clean Eating (and Living)

- **Take a Mental Health Fast**

Take a spiritual, mental-health day (or week). Turn off the television; put your newspaper subscription on hold for a week; go entirely off-line. Too much all at once? Try one abstention at a time: a news fast or a verbal austerity gossip-free fast. Turn off your BlackBerry on Sundays. Don't answer the phone after 8 P.M. a couple of evenings a week. Take a weekend off from social plans. Avoid violent movies and television shows. Skip the celebrity news magazine for a week or two or, even better, take a break from toxic relationships and find some spiritual soul mates. As Swami Prabhavananda and Christopher Isherwood put it in *How to Know God*, "cultivate the society of those who are spiritually minded."

- **Have a Light Eating Day**

Pick one day a week when you're less active than usual to go especially light on your eating. I first encountered this idea in Dr. Andrew Weil's books, before realizing that fasting and light eating are a part of many spiritual and religious traditions (Yom Kippur, Ramadan, Lent). Not that it has to be so serious or ascetic; think of this as a "spa cuisine" day—a treat you can give yourself. Maybe you'll decide to have a fruit-and-vegetable-only day; or you'll stick to clean foods like brown rice and salmon and steamed kale and chard. See it as a pleasure rather than a punishment to give your digestive system a break. For her light-eating days, my friend Daphne likes to make a pot of simple vegetable broth and have it over the course of several mealtimes. Try sipping this with some "tricked-out" water—not the ultra-processed vitamin water sold in stores (which doesn't do much for you nutritionally) but filtered tap water to which you add slices of thoroughly washed organic lemon or lime. Yogis in the know claim that the lemon and lime will help cleanse your system. It's essential on a light-eating day but great anytime.

• What About Cleanses?

Having lived in Los Angeles, I couldn't help but run into yogis who have done, and loved, The Master Cleanse—a fasting regimen involving maple syrup, cayenne pepper, and fresh lemon juice. I have friends, too, who've successfully tried some less-stringent (and crazy-sounding) fasts, like a yeast-free fast, with good results. Use your common sense, and don't feel like you have to buy an expensive cleansing package or system to purify your diet. Eating clean and light can be done cheaply and simply by cutting out things like animal products, processed foods, and dairy—and adding in more fruits and vegetables and whole grains. Save the maple syrup for the (very) occasional, homemade, whole wheat pancakes!

Daphne's Broth

One package of organic vegetable broth (or make fresh if you like!)

2 cloves garlic, sliced

1 teaspoon grated fresh ginger

1 or 2 small green chili peppers (Indian or jalapeño)

1 stalk celery, coarsely sliced (or just use the leftover leafy ends of a few stalks)

2 or 3 carrots, coarsely sliced

Add all to broth and bring to a simmer. Add the garlic, ginger, and celery. Cook for 15 minutes on low heat and strain if desired—or go ahead and eat everything but the peppers.

7

nonviolence (ahimsa)

*MAY ALL BEINGS EVERYWHERE
BE HAPPY AND FREE—INCLUDING YOU
(AHIMSA: NONHARMING, NONVIOLENCE)*

*SUTRA II.35: AHIMSAPRATISTHAYAM
TATSANNIDAU VAIRATYAGAH*

The more considerate one is, the more one stimulates friendly feelings among all in one's presence. —T. K. V. Desikachar

May All Beings Everywhere Be Happy and Free

Meat eaters take a deep, yogic breath: I'm about to talk about vegetarianism. For many yogis, vegetarianism follows from the concept of *ahimsa* or nonviolence. Yoga expert Geeta Iyengar writes in her book, *Yoga: A Gem for Women*: "[V]iolence is lack of love . . . A yogi has no hatred in the heart, but only love for all. Nonviolence is respect for others; it is a state of mind. Patañjali says [in the Sutras] that anyone coming into contact with a yogi who is devoid of thoughts of violence is bound to cast off feelings of enmity."

FEATURED POSE: Cobbler's Pose (*Baddha Konasana*)

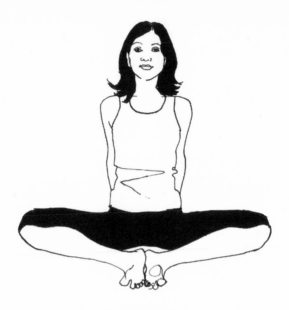

Sit on one or two neatly folded blankets. Bring your feet together so that the insides of the feet are touching and allow
your knees to open and release to either side. If this is difficult—as it may well be—sit up on more height, and place
padding underneath the knees on either side. You can also set
yourself up in this pose with your back against a wall for extra support. Breathing into the hips, release them further and
further down. With your hands, open your feet like pages in a
book; this will further open the hips. Practicing this pose for
several minutes each day will not only transform your pose by
opening your hips, it will also change the way your body feels
and moves in the world.

In the presence of one firmly established in non-violence, all hostilities cease.

—Sri Swami Satchidananda

I first learned about the concept of *ahimsa* at the Jivamukti Yoga Center, where vegetarianism is considered more beautiful than any yoga pose. My favorite Jivamukti teacher Ruth said that nonviolence had to do not just with the big decisions in life, but the smallest of actions, too. The best and simplest way to practice nonviolence, according to Ruth, and Jivamukti founders Sharon Gannon and David Life, is to become a vegetarian.

Before class we'd chant, "May all beings everywhere be happy and free" in Sanskrit—*Lokah Samasta Sukhino Bhavantu*—and discuss what this means. Our teachers reminded us, gently, that *ahimsa* means we need to be kind to one another, work toward a world where everyone has enough to eat and a safe and warm place to live and raise their family—*and* to think of our animal friends and stop eating them.

At that time I was twenty-six, and I'd lost some of the good eating habits I'd picked up in Nepal, along with the pure vegetarianism I'd adopted abroad. I liked the idea of *ahimsa* when it came to humans—who wouldn't?—but the animal aspect didn't resonate with me in the same way. Who had time to think about animals? There were too many other things wrong with the world. And besides, I was too busy fighting for my own survival: I had a career to establish, rent to make, graduate school applications to fill out, the love of my life to find.

A Yogi has no hatred in the heart, but only love for all. Violence is the outcome of fear, selfishness, anger, and lack of confidence. Non-violence is respect for others; it is a state of mind.

—Geeta Iyengar

"May all beings everywhere be happy and free." It's a beautiful prayer, one that grows on you, taking on different and deeper meanings the more you chant it. May *all* beings *everywhere* be happy and free—a prayer for all living things, no matter how celebrated or humble. Over time, the message sunk in. In the years that followed, I gradually worked on eliminating meat and poultry from my diet, making my meals more consistent with the principles of *ahimsa*. These days, I'm a fish vegetarian. I'm far from an icon of nonviolent perfection—salmon are living beings, too, after all—but I'm working on having my choices around food be gentler on the planet, and on my family's health.

Meat Is Murder?

Giving up meat isn't as big a deal as it may sound. I have to tell you that I don't miss it at all, and for those of you who like your steak or bacon or chicken teriyaki, I'll bet my hemp-seed eye pillow that the more you eat in an enlightened way, the less meat you'll crave, too. Being a vegetarian doesn't need to feel like a deprivation. Between tofu, lentils, beans, whole grains, fruits and vegetables, organic dairy products, and the occasional piece of fish, I have a wide range of primary ingredients to choose from. I've traveled through Europe and Asia and not felt overly constrained by my choices. Sure, there are some dishes I have to avoid, and certain tastes I have to give up. But the truth is that staying healthy and thin means being reasonably careful about what you eat no matter what. Being a vegetarian, I like not having to worry about the inadvertently gristly or bloody bite or having to clean and prepare old cuts of a dead animal in my kitchen and worry about salmonella and mixing meat- and veggie-friendly cutting boards. My food tastes better to me knowing that no animals were killed in the process of bringing the meal to the table.

As much as I love being a vegetarian, and think you will, too, I'm not going to *insist* on your going cold turkey (so to speak). There are many ways to practice *ahimsa*; how we treat our fellow humans, for starters, is enough to keep us occupied for several lifetimes. And the yogi doesn't shy away from moral complexity, preferring flexibility over rigid stances. Consider the words of the yoga scholar and philosopher T. K. V. Desikachar, who asks:

> [S]hould we as vegetarians find ourselves in a situation where there is only meat to eat, is it better to starve to death than to eat what is there? If we still have something to do in this life, such as family responsibilities, then we should avoid doing anything that may cause us harm or prevent us from carrying out our duties. The answer in this situation is clear— it would show a lack of consideration and arrogance to become stuck on our principles. . . . In every situation we should adopt a considered attitude. That is the meaning of *ahimsa*.

Still, being enlightened, spiritually and nutritionally healthy, in my opinion, does require that you cut down—a lot—on your meat and poultry consumption.

Strong Island

When I was a kid, eating meat was a given. A well-rounded meal in my house in the 1970s and 1980s—and maybe yours too—centered around some kind of animal protein, say ground beef or chicken, with frozen vegetables, maybe string beans or peas or carrots, on the side. For an especially festive family dinner, we'd do taco night—ground beef and shredded cheese in a corn taco shell with a little lettuce on top. In the summer, we'd grill burgers and hot dogs on the barbecue in the backyard. On Sunday mornings, my dad made pancakes or eggs and served them with sausage links. Eating out mostly meant McDonald's or pizza. On a special occasion, we'd head out to the Chinese restaurant in town, decorated in red lacquer with signed and framed New York Islander hockey team photos, for pepper steak, moo shoo pork, chicken and broccoli, and fried egg rolls. Sometimes, on Saturday nights, my parents hired a babysitter and we got to stay up late watching a triple feature of *Solid Gold*, *The Love Boat*, and *Fantasy Island* after eating our TV dinners of turkey with cranberry sauce or Salisbury steak. We were *lucky* to be able to eat meat most nights, my mom reminded us.

As I think back on it, I was a somewhat reluctant meat eater. Many kids are. Anthropologists Marvin Harris and Eric B. Ross, drawing on a number of different studies, argue that most food preferences—including the taste for meat—are learned, not innate. (On the other hand, researchers note, kids *do* inherently like sweets. Maybe that explains Lucien's love of yogurt and fruit.) The taste of meat, however, isn't always a natural one, and to me the idea of eating those cute cows we'd spot on the side of the road or on school field trips to the farms in the further outreaches of Long Island seemed wrong, and kind of gross.

"Don't you know where that comes from?" I'd ask my brothers, pointing at their plates.

"Jessie, eat your dinner," my mother pleaded.

Often I would. Too often, according to the bathroom scale. Not knowing what my vegetarian options were—more bagels and french fries and extra cheese pizza? Iceberg lettuce with croutons and salad dressing?—I did what I was told. Ignoring my vegetarian intuition, I'd order a really well-done, beyond-burnt, cheeseburger deluxe platter at the diner. Or I'd have the $5 chicken and broccoli dish that came with soup and orange slices—the one my friend Kathy (the same friend who twenty years later told me to walk after my C-section) and I would eat for lunch at the Chinese restaurant in town. Another favorite was the beef negimaki (thinly rolled slices of beef with saucy, salty scallions) that we served at the Japanese restaurant where I worked. God help me, I even loved the chicken sandwich at Burger King.

Holy Cows

In Nepal I first started to understand how you could not just survive, but thrive, on a vegetarian diet. There, both for religious reasons (cows are considered holy beings) and for financial ones (meat is prohibitively expensive for people living on a dollar a day) vegetarian meals are the rule rather than the exception. During homestays and at village teahouses and Katmandu restaurants, I was treated to a ridiculously tasty menu of vegetables, legumes, spices, and grains.

After my semester in Nepal, I worked on a kibbutz in Israel, both in the fields and in the kitchen, where I helped harvest and prepare fresh local foods. I picked buckets of apples, and peeled and chopped barrels of beets and potatoes and buckets of cucumbers. Though the secular kibbutz kitchen wasn't vegetarian (or kosher), it was vegetarian-friendly. I learned a lot that summer about how to fill up my plate and my diet with foods other than meat.

I kept up with my fledgling vegetarianism for a while but went on and off the chuck wagon, lured by a tempting side order of bacon with my eggs at a diner after a weekend of camping; a cheeseburger and beer with a new boyfriend; or strips of grilled chicken on my salad, which I hoped would help me lose weight.

Martha's Co-op

When I was accepted into a housing cooperative called Martha's during my graduate-school days, I gave up meat for good. Martha's was a big, old, collectively-owned ramshackle house on a lake a short walk from campus. The rent was super-cheap, and to supplement our financial contribution, those of us who lived there had to do several hours per week of work around the house, everything from cooking and cleaning to babysitting and insulating windows in wintertime.

The hub of Martha's was the kitchen. It was there, amid the mismatched and decades-old sets of dishes and pots and pans, that thirty adults and a handful of members' children gathered each night for dinner. As part of our work responsibilities, we took turns making dinner for the house, baking bread, and cleaning up after meals. We were on our own for breakfast and lunch, but even those turned out to be communal experiences. When you made your way down to the colorfully painted kitchen with its long wooden table, you'd usually find a housemate cooking up a tofu scramble or a veggie melt sandwich on whole wheat bread or pouring a bowl of organic Puffins cereal, popping popcorn or baking oatmeal cookies or scoring the last piece of fruit from the counter by the window.

Martha's was strictly vegetarian. Fish was forbidden—even dairy was contentious. Some of our members were Midwestern-born meat eaters, others punk-style vegans, but in order to live together in relatively crunchy harmony, we compromised on a vegetarian meal plan with vegan options at dinnertime. The tastiness depended on who was doing the cooking on any given night, but I do remember some delicious meals: whole wheat pasta with fresh-from-the-farm vegetables, sautéed tofu squares with home-baked beans and quinoa, veggie burgers and kale. Once again, I came to see how easy, cheap, and delicious eating vegetarian could be.

Six Reasons Not to Eat Meat

1. Reduce your carbon footprint without having to plunk down the money for a new Prius.
2. Lose weight without really trying.
3. Lower your grocery bills without really trying, too.
4. Tofu is the new chicken.
5. Automatically up your hipster quotient.
6. Veggie burgers with guacamole, tomato, and onion. YUM.

The Sad Cows on Highway 5

For those of you who *are* going to keep eating meat, you can still practice *ahimsa* by eating animals that are raised humanely. There really is a difference. I didn't realize how poorly we treat our livestock animals until Neil and I took a long drive from Los Angeles to the San Francisco Bay Area, where Neil grew up. We were somewhere in the middle of California, when, all of the sudden, the smell hit me. Thousands upon thousands of sad-looking cows were packed into claustrophobic pastures. The cows were everywhere, stuffed into never-ending fields on either side of the highway, crowded beyond belief, the stench of their colossally cramped quarters hanging in the air like a toxic cloud.

"Don't look!" Neil said, covering my eyes with his right hand as he drove. But I pushed him away. This I had to see for myself. It's one thing to raise animals humanely for meat. Here was something altogether different—an animal prison, a torture chamber, a living hell. Suddenly the animal-loving girl in me who refused to dissect a frog in the ninth grade was shaken awake.

At least those cows were able to walk outside. Most hens, pregnant sows, and veal calves spend their lives in cramped pens, never getting to see the sun or feel fresh air or turn around or spread their wings or limbs before being slaughtered.

Have you seen the footage of lambs chained to their stalls by the neck? Once you do, I promise you'll never look at a plate of non-free-range meat the same way again. Thankfully, animal practices are starting to change. In November 2008, Proposition 2 passed in California, requiring that animals have at least a little more room in their stalls and pens. In the U.K., there's a widely supported movement toward more-humane treatment of livestock and, more generally, organic farming practices. Sadly, though, most of the animals raised for meat these days live more like the animals on Highway 5 than like those we picture in our bucolic images of life on the farm.

Happy as CSA Pigs

Things can be different. Some animals *do* have the chance to lead decent, maybe even enlightened, lives before heading off to the chopping block. I believe that farmers who treat animals with dignity and grace, letting them roam fields freely and nurse at their mothers' breasts, practice *ahimsa* in their animal husbandry. This means that buying meat produced from ethically raised and farmed livestock is a meaningful consumer choice, the meat eater's *ahimsa*. From what I hear from my meat-eating friends, free-range meat tastes better, too.

During our year in the country, Neil and I joined a Community Supported Agriculture (CSA) farm. Each week

when Neil and I went to pick up—and in some cases, pick—
our weekly allotment of seasonal veggies and fruit and drop
off our compost bucket, we'd stop to admire and coo at the
baby pigs in the barn. And then one late-October day, the
kind of day that makes you dig out your woolens from winter storage, we drove out to the farm for what would be one
of the last times before the snow and frost hit. We filled up
our crate with fall vegetables and grabbed a pumpkin for our
porch. The pigs, our usual stop on the way to stocking up on
garlic and onions from the bins in the barn, were gone, their
stalls cleaned out. At the cashier's table, people were paying
for their cuts of pork.

Poor pigs, we said. I flashed back to watching *Charlotte's
Web* and the scene where Wilbur the piglet nursed from his
bottle in Fern's lap. But deep down I knew how much the
farmers and their interns had loved those pigs, had treated
them with tenderness and care, and had given them a beautiful setting in which to live. These animals had lived very
different lives from the cows we'd seen in California.

Pony Up

Even if you do buy free-range, ethically produced meat,
I still recommend eating less of it. One way to do this is
to marry your ethical meat eating with a Nepali sensibility
toward meat—making meat a special-occasion-only food,

using it to garnish and flavor your dishes rather than as the main event on your plate seven days a week. In his important book, *In Defense of Food*, Michael Pollan writes that "eating a little meat isn't going to kill you, though it might be better approached as a side dish than as a main."

How to Eat Less Meat

- **Work Your Way Down the Animal Kingdom**

Take a gradual approach. Begin by cutting out beef, then move on to ban pork and lamb, and then nix poultry from your diet. (Beef has been linked to an increased risk of some cancers, and has a particularly large environmental impact.)

- **Eat More Fish**

This might sound counter-intuitive—and not very compassionate to our fish friends—but subbing fish for meat can work wonders in easing the transition from meat eating to vegetarianism. Whether you can't imagine a meal without an animal protein, or can't find something strictly vegetarian to order when eating out at a restaurant, a piece of salmon (preferably wild, not farmed), or a shrimp dish, can save the day. Sushi, for example, is a tasty and healthy way to enjoy a meal out—as long as you avoid the "special" rolls containing tempura or high fat, mayonnaise-based sauces. And, while of course fish are living beings, it does feel different to think about eating a fish than a walking, squawking fowl or moo-ing mammal. Fish oils are great for your skin and hair, too. Don't go overboard (ha-ha) with fish, though. It's important to be conscious of mercury levels in seafood. (Fish with lower mercury content include trout, scallops, salmon, and tilapia.

Tuna, halibut, and swordfish tend to have high mercury levels.) But eating more fish is a great way to get started living meat-free.

• A Rose By Any Other Name . . .

Call your animal products what they are. A steak is a slice of cow, a pork loin is flesh from a pig's ribcage area. A tongue, is, well, a tongue. If you're still hungry for meat after reframing your menu non-euphemistically, at least you're being honest with yourself—and the animal on your plate.

The benefits of reducing your meat intake are related to both health and environment. Marion Nestle writes that "the meat industry's big public relations problem is that vegetarians are demonstrably healthier than meat eaters. If you do not eat beef, pork, lamb, or even chicken, your risk of heart disease and certain cancers is likely to be lower than that of the average meat-eating American." At the same time, a vegetarian, or mostly vegetarian, diet is good for the planet's health, too. Raising animals for meat leaves an incredibly large carbon footprint. In his book *Food Matters*, the *New York Times* food columnist Mark Bittman writes that, according to a recent United Nations report, "Gobal livestock production is responsible for about one-fifth of all greenhouse gases—more than transportation. . . . Another way to put it is that eating a typical family-of-four steak dinner is the rough equivalent, energy-wise, of driving around in an SUV for three hours while leaving all the lights on at home." Unbelievable, isn't it?

Look, I know that adopting a vegetarian diet can be a big, identity-changing step. What we eat is about more than just calories and taste and nutrition; it's about family and ritual and culture, too. For me, forever a Jewish girl from suburban Long Island, my deepest meat memory is my grandmother's two-day pot roast. For you it might be fried chicken, or your dad's meatloaf, a pepperoni pizza, a sticky-on-the-bottom paella with sausage, or a holiday ham.

At Martha's Co-op, every couple of months there'd be a showdown at our Sunday-night house meetings between the vegetarians and the meat eaters. The skinny, hippie, and hipster vegetarians were sometimes in danger of being overthrown from power by animal-protein-craving, meat-loving insurgents. A favorite argument during these meetings was that vegetarianism is classist and racist: classist, because not everyone can afford to eat vegetarian, and racist, because it requires people to abandon their traditional food ways and start acting like privileged white college kids in Berkeley, California (or Poughkeepsie, New York—or Madison, Wisconsin, for that matter). I got what my housemates and friends were saying and share their concerns about culture and class and food, but I don't buy their conclusions.

As for money, it's true that nothing is as convenient and cheap as a dollar meal at McDonald's. But (a) once you get your vegetarian kitchen up and running, the average vegetarian meal will cost you half as much to prepare as the average meat meal; and (b) heart disease and other obesity-related illnesses extract too high a financial, not to mention emotional, price for their ease and convenience. Want a dollar meal? Try one of our favorite quick, cheap, and easy dinners. We started making this, and then one day a Latina cashier at a Brooklyn corner store told us her family eats it all the time too: brown rice and black beans, mixed together with a bit of grated cheese and a generous splash of hot sauce. The rice and beans together give you what nutritionists call a complete protein, and if you add some Swiss chard or kale sautéed in a bit of olive oil on the side, you've got a perfect dinner that'll only cost you a few dollars—and maybe even less—per serving.

Besides, spending a little more on food—for organics, or for wild fish, for example—will most likely save you (and the economy at large) money on health-care costs later on. Experts agree that our Western diet is making us sick—from heart disease to diabetes to cancer. Real, whole, unprocessed, healthful foods are an essential part of life, and worth spending money on; much more so than any clothing or electronics you might buy. You're *worth* the investment. As Michael Pollan points out, "Traditionally people have allocated a far greater proportion of their income to food—as they still do in several of the countries where people eat better than we do, and as a consequence are healthier than we are."

As for the convenience of fast food, it's true you'll have a hard time finding a drive-through tofu stand, but if you dig around your town or city, chances are you'll find a few vegetarian (or vegetarian-friendly) restaurants.

The cultural tradition argument, for its part, is a bit of a red herring—or perhaps a gefilte fish. So many of the consumption practices we think of as traditional, my sociologist husband Neil likes to remind me, were either invented relatively recently or have already been substantially modified to adapt to modern conditions. For instance, as historian Stephanie Coontz explains in her book, *The Way We Never Were: American Families and the Nostalgia Trap*, the idea of a nuclear family with a male breadwinner and stay-at-home mother is a relatively recent construct that became solidified in the national imagination in the 1950s. Before that, especially for working-class families, it was very common for both adults to participate in the labor force. In much the same way, many foods we consider to be culturally meaningful are newer inventions than you might think, much as the modern-day Christmas tree is from Germany, not Jerusalem. Point being, you and your cultural traditions *can* adapt and be flexible enough to make room for a more vegetarian sensibility.

But there are other reasons besides cost and tradition that might deter you from embracing an all or mostly veggie diet. Maybe you feel like your family and friends won't accept you as a vegetarian. And what will you do when traveling and exploring other countries, cultures, or even just at a friend's place for dinner, when meat is what's offered? Maybe you've had some early tragic experiences with tofu. (My husband almost ruined tofu forever for our baby by serving it to him one rushed afternoon, straight out of the fridge with no preparation at all. Yes, tofu *is* disgusting when served raw.) Some of us just need a couple of really convincing meat-free meals—a perfectly made lentil veggie burger with yam fries, for example, or an off-the-hook Indian feast. Others will need to go through a deeper process of self-exploration.

Neil's Story

Neil's a good example of type B. When we met he was an unapologetic meat eater who loved nothing more than a good burger or some barbecued ribs. These days he's a dyed-in-the-100-percent-wool vegetarian who can't imagine how he ever ate meat on a daily basis. Neil grew up in a close-knit three-person family, the only child of a very loving and attentive mother and father in Berkeley, California. To them, good food almost always meant meat. Neil's mother even self-published a cookbook in the early 1980s called *Cooking for the Way We Live Today*, filled with beef, chicken, and pork recipes ready for quick preparation in the food processor. She and Neil's father were part of a gourmet club that exchanged recipes and held dinner parties where meat was always on the menu. On very special occasions, they dined at Alice Waters's famous Berkeley farm-to-table restaurant, Chez Panisse.

Tragically, Neil lost both of his parents when he was in his twenties. After Neil's mom died of cancer, his dad ate out more, gaining more weight with each passing year. When, almost a decade later, Neil's father died of a heart attack related to being overweight, Neil broke down and grieved in a soul-searching, life-altering way. At the age of twenty-nine, he started rethinking everything about his life—including his relationship with food.

If only subconsciously, Neil had always equated meat with not only his parents and his childhood but also with a certain type of manliness, too. He'd worked as a police officer for a year after college. Eating bacon and eggs and drinking scotch with the guys after pulling a night shift was as much a part of the scene as stopping for donuts and coffee or being a gym rat on days off.

Neil was with his father on the day he died. Right or wrong, he started associating meat with his father's death—the sad particulars of the greasy pork lunch he'd had that day and, more generally, his father's "life is meant to be enjoyed" philosophy around food. Neil stopped equating meat with masculinity. After a particularly gristly hamburger one day in our Brooklyn neighborhood, he gave up meat altogether and didn't look back.

Once he became a vegetarian, he lost a good twenty pounds without dieting at all and became a lithe yoga type. And as I've mentioned, Neil doesn't actually *do* much yoga. Even after all these years together, I have to plead with him—or drag him—to get him to take a yoga class. He loves it once he goes, but he's always got a ridiculously long to-do list at work and more than a full plate at home between being a good husband and father. With his vegetarian diet, though, he *looks* like someone who gets his downward dog on five days a week. His meat-eating friends are always asking him for his secret—how has he escaped the dreaded midlife paunch? The answer is, more than anything, because he's a vegetarian (and most meat is fattening and artery-clogging)!

Make the decision to eat less meat. Don't do it just for the animals or because you're concerned about global warming (both great reasons); do it for you, because you'll feel healthier with a more plant-based diet. As Michael Pollan puts it, "Eat food. Not too much. Mostly plants." (Sounds a lot like Ram Dass, doesn't he?)

What's the Deal with Vegans?

Spend any time among yogis, and you'll quickly discover there are as many kinds of vegetarians as there are colors of Havaiana flip-flops lining the halls of Los Angeles yoga centers. Some who would describe themselves as vegetarians abstain only from red meat, while others eschew meat and poultry, as well as fish. The ultra-orthodox of vegetarians are vegans—people who also eliminate animal by-products from their diet, avoiding eggs, cheese, milk, and all other dairy products. When it comes to clothes and accessories, vegans usually reject wearing leather or other animal skins, too. (My ex-boyfriend's sisters opened up a vegan shoe store in downtown Manhattan to offer fashionable footwear for their fellow believers.) Consider any movement you can make toward vegetarianism, small or large, as a positive step toward physical and karmic health.

Check out *Skinny Bitch* by Rory Freedman and Kim Barnouin for more on vegan eating and the director of the Jivamukti Yoga Center Sharon Gannon's book, *Yoga and Vegetarianism*, for more on the relationship between *ahimsa* and a vegetarian diet.

8

self-study and introspection (svadhyaya)

READY, SET, MEDITATE

(SVADHYAYA: SELF-STUDY)
SUTRA II.44: *SVADHYAYAT ISTADEVATA SAMPRAYOGAH*

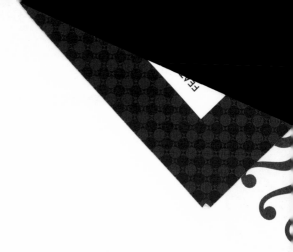

Self-study leads toward the
realization of God or communion with
one's desired deity. —B. K. S. Iyengar

You can work out on the treadmill for as long as you
like, eat apples and cauliflower heads for dinner, and
lose all the weight you want, but until you take the time to
do some serious internal work, you probably won't be able to
bring about the kind of lasting life changes you're craving. We
all have psychic scars that need healing—emotional wounds
from our early years that remain open. It's these traumas and
fears that lay behind so much overeating. Coming to know
yourself better through self-study and introspection so that
you can make progress with these emotional issues is the key
to keeping the weight off, and to setting yourself on a deeper
spiritual path.

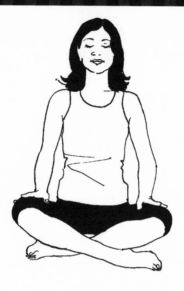

Sit on a folded blanket or two so that your hips are higher than your knees, in a cross-legged position. Place your ankles underneath your knees and rest your hands on your thighs. If it's difficult for you to sit this way for more than a minute or two, begin by sitting on a chair. The important thing is to be in a position where you can be still. Breathe in and out, slowly and consciously, through your nose, allowing your chest to fill up with breath and then empty out again. Relax your jaw. Let go of your thoughts, if you can do so without causing anxiety. Or else, allow your mind to follow your thoughts without worry or judgment. Try to remain here for two or three to five minutes in the beginning, slowly working your way up to ten or even twenty or thirty minutes a day. As my former teacher Baron Baptiste says, "Let go, and let God."

The more effective our study, the more we understand our weaknesses and our strengths. We learn to nullify our weaknesses and use our strengths to the utmost. Then there is no limit to our understanding.

—T. K. V. Desikachar

A place to begin is by acknowledging your pain or anger. What have you been through? How much hurt have you endured? Who, if anyone, was to blame? And what did you have to do to survive? Whether you're mad at yourself, your parents, your current or former partners, or even with God, the challenge now is to start coming to terms with your past so that you can move forward into a happier, healthier future. How can this be more than New Age, feel-good mumbo jumbo? The answer revolves around forgiveness, something that was difficult for me to contemplate after I stopped talking to my parents. Remember the sutra I quoted in chapter one: Undisturbed calmness of mind is attained by cultivating friendliness toward the happy, compassion for the unhappy, delight in the virtuous, and indifference toward the wicked. "We must practice indifference toward the hurts we receive from others," Swami Prabhavananda and Christopher Isherwood continue. "We must go behind the wickedness of the wicked and try to understand what makes them treat us that way."

What I learned, eventually, was that forgiveness doesn't mean we must reconcile with those who have wronged us (I've chosen to remain estranged from my parents). The only must is to open our eyes to the humanness of all, including those who have caused us pain and suffering, and acknowledge the hard times they faced that led them to behave as they did toward us. For me, this meant coming to understand that the physical abuse my father suffered as a child led him to repeat the pattern. Forgiveness means no more than this sort of understanding; it's the first step toward healing, because it removes the unhealthy mental energy we tend to devote to people who (and experiences which) have caused us trauma. The yogi is practical and action-oriented and forgives, because to forgive is to free oneself from suffering.

Forgiveness relates to weight loss directly through the notion of what yogis call *samskaras*. These are the habits and engrained patterns we tend to fall back on when experiencing stress or pain. A negative *samskara* can be anything from the cigarette you light up to the junk food you reach for when you're sad to the tendency to be quick to anger when provoked. What the yogi tries to do is replace bad habits with good ones, to create new and life-affirming *samskaras*. Healing, forgiveness, and making peace with our past creates the mental space for this to happen, and makes it less likely we'll revert to bad habits. When it comes to food and exercise, the goal is to get rid of negative *samskaras*—a sedentary lifestyle, for example, or a taste for fried and processed foods, or the idea that eating a rich dessert every night is "normal"—so that you can build a new and improved life.

Pause for a big grain of sea salt: I'm no guru on a mountaintop, and I have as many bad habits and negative *samskaras* as the next person. I anger quickly; I get sad easily; I can be greedy, too often thinking about myself first and others second. I can be too hard on myself. (See previous sentence.) The only way that I can imagine moving beyond my shortcomings is to become aware of them—to study myself and work on becoming more even-keeled, more loving, more generous, more self-aware.

For me, this has involved therapy; study of spiritual books; finding friendship and community with other seekers; spending more time in nature, meditation, yoga, and community service; taking part in chanting sessions; mothering, teaching, writing, and being a friend; and day-to-day living in a conscious and evolving relationship with Neil. And then, there's something that's always been harder for me to talk about—my personal, not always easy, relationship with something deeper . . . with God.

The companion piece to self-knowledge is getting in touch with a higher power, whether a personal God or a more diffuse force like nature. Surrender and devotion, yogis believe, brings freedom from suffering. You may choose to pray in a church or synagogue or mosque, perform *puja* (worship) at a temple altar, walk through a forest or on a beach, or, most simply, close your eyes and listen to your breath.

Om Shanti

I've always liked the idea of meditation. As a girl, I remember thinking there was something almost romantic about sitting so still. For a long time, though, I needed something (a mountain) or someone (a yoga teacher) to take me to that peaceful place of oneness. Just sitting? I couldn't do it. I'd been told that in meditation you're supposed to close your eyes and "let go" of your thoughts, to have them come "in one ear, and out the other." But whenever I tried to meditate by myself, my thoughts raced in place right where they were, staying firmly stuck in my brain, smack dab between my ears. After a minute or two, I'd give up.

All we require, at the beginning, is a seed. And the seed need be nothing more than a feeling of interest in the possibilities of the spiritual life.

—Swami Prabhavananda and
Christopher Isherwood

So I tried organized sittings. For a while Neil and I attended a weekly meditation group in L.A. led by a psychology professor who was a Buddhist. His instructions were different; rather than trying to shut down our thoughts, he said we should follow them, watch them, and then, when the meditation was done, share the stream of consciousness that flooded through us with other members of the group. We didn't even have to sit up in a classic meditation posture, he said. We could sit on a couch, on the floor, or even lay in bed.

Then there was a day-long meditation retreat at a center in Marin County, California. Our teacher led us in a sitting in a light-filled hall and then sent us outside to the grounds where we walked in a circular walking meditation. The movement helped me concentrate on each new moment. Years later, at another meditation center, this time in Boston, I managed to sit still for a long while and felt something like what I'd experienced on mountaintops in Nepal. Slowly, very slowly, my mind quieted.

Still, it seemed, I needed to attend a class or retreat in order to meditate. Meditating on my own on a daily basis seemed infinitely harder than any handstand or headstand. Then, a few years ago, on assignment for a magazine, I attended a workshop on restorative yoga with Judith Lasater, a well-known and highly respected senior teacher. Restorative yoga is heaven: Wearing sweats and wool socks, we spent two blissful hours in various forms of rest—with our legs up the wall or on our backs with pillows propping every possible body part. After we'd finished the poses, Judith discussed the importance of having a daily restorative practice—even if that means just a five-minute corpse pose, or *savasana*, before bed—*and* a daily meditation practice. In the question-and-answer period, I asked what her advice might be for someone like me who wanted to meditate but was having a hard time getting into a routine.

"Start with two minutes," Judith said. "And then, five, and then for a long, long while, ten. And eventually, twenty." This advice may sound basic, but for me it was a revelation. Before this, anything less than a twenty-minute sitting had seemed like a failure. But, like a headstand, a meditation practice has to be built up minute by minute. I did what she suggested. Following Dr. Lasater's instructions, I simply sat in bed on a pillow as soon as I got up in the morning, even before peeing. (If I got up to go to the bathroom, I knew I'd talk myself out of meditating and get pulled into my morning routine of coffee and the computer and e-mail and work.) I used a small digital clock to tick off the minutes and placed a still sleepy Salem at my feet. Why Salem? It helped to have a silent partner in the ritual. Sometimes I'd massage her while meditating and that helped me, too. I'd set the alarm for however many minutes I was up to, close my eyes, and breathe. It didn't take much time—only a few months—to gradually go from two to twenty minutes. When I backtracked and missed a few days, which happened often, I'd begin the cycle again.

When I became anxious or depressed or worried, those morning minutes brought me back to myself. Getting started with meditation can sometimes be anxiety-producing—we aren't used to being so inwardly focused—but, in time, my meditation became a deeply calming and centering experience. It will become that for you, too. When you find that you can become your own source of contentment and calm, you won't need to indulge in unhealthy habits like overeating to fill up that emotional space inside. Meditation not only helped me stay healthy and thin, but also made it possible for me to continue to live depression-free. I came to see that there was a place in me that nobody, not even my parents, were able to damage, a place that was whole and perfect.

To be honest, meditation is *still* a struggle—not so much sitting still anymore (by now I like the silence) but just finding the time to do it. With a baby in the house, not to mention a book to write, some days I'm happy to find the time to change out of my pajamas. And many days I need any free time I can get to do a simple yoga pose, reply to an e-mail, make myself something to eat, bathe. (Those of you with multiple children and/or high-stress careers and commutes don't need me to tell you any of this.)

Still, no matter *what* our household and work obligations, if we want to meditate, if we long for that kind of daily peace and stillness, we've just got to make the time. Maybe it's the moment before you start your car or while on the bus to work in the morning. Maybe you can meditate in the shower. Or maybe you can take a couple of minutes to sit up in bed in the morning and breathe in and out.

Now that Lucien is a year old, and I'm finally catching up on my sleep, my plan is to dust off my alarm clock, rally my meditation partner, Salem, and begin building a daily meditation practice once again. I'll start slow, with two minutes, and then five and then ten and then, eventually, twenty. Maybe one day, when I'm a silver-haired eighty-year-old yogi, I'll be able to sit for an hour or two on a mountaintop, or bask in the sun in the middle of my garden.

On the Couch

Another form of self-study is therapy. As with yoga asana practice or meditation, who you study with matters. Battling depression on and off during my adolescence and twenties, I tried counseling sessions here and there, but they weren't very helpful. Eventually, thanks to some good health coverage, I found two great therapists—in different parts of the country, at different critical junctures in my life. Both were older, wiser women who were part spiritual guide and part maternal figure. My therapists helped me deal with the aftermath of the decision to separate from my parents, and inspired me to dream big—to believe that I could be happy.

With the right therapist, therapy and making the change to healthy eating and exercise can go hand in hand. Mine helped me figure out what I was eating that was making me gain and keep on weight and why I was eating that way despite how it made me look and feel. To end my struggle with obesity, I needed to delve into the cobwebbed and closed-off places in my psyche, places that were painful but necessary to revisit.

Out in the World

Self-knowledge can also be directed outward. With it, you can become a source of good and light in the world. Yogis often dedicate their spiritual practice to something beyond themselves. As you become healthier and happier, you'll naturally turn your focus to the world outside your door, the world that needs your help. You'll find small and, later, larger ways to use your new clearer, lighter bodies and minds to help others—volunteering, helping an elderly neighbor or taking on a cause like hunger or poverty or literacy or access to health care.

For starters, by becoming a little bit more enlightened, you'll automatically become an example and a role model to family members, friends, and coworkers hoping to make their own positive, healthy lifestyle changes. You'll inspire them to eat better and exercise more. You don't need to get out your megaphone and start preaching. Just like Jackie, Jenna, Leigh, and so many other friends—and teachers—in my life helped me by gently, quietly, and lovingly nudging me along my path, you'll do the same for those in your life.

9

touching enlightenment
(santosa, samadhi)

GO AHEAD, YOU KNOW YOU WANT TO

(SANTOSA: CONTENTMENT)
SUTRA II.42: *SANTOSAT ANUTTAMAH SUKHALABHAH*

(SAMADHI: PURE CONSCIOUSNESS, BLISS)

SUTRA II.45: *SAMADHISIDDHIH ISVARAPRANIDHANAT*

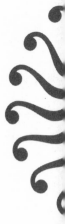

The result of contentment is total happiness. The happiness we get from acquiring passions is only temporary. We need to find new ones and acquire them to sustain this sort of happiness. There is no end to it. But true contentment, leading to total happiness and bliss, is in a class by itself. —T. K. V. Desikachar

We moved around a lot after our year in the Berkshires. Neil found a job in Los Angeles and then another in Boston. In Massachusetts, I studied Iyengar yoga, and learned more about how to integrate the Sutras into my daily life, with the renowned senior teacher Patricia Walden.

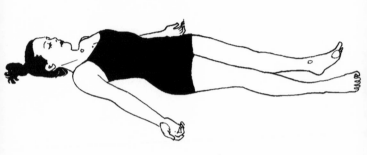

Lie on the floor, on your back. (If this feels uncomfortable, place a yoga bolster, or a rolled blanket, underneath your knees.) Rest your arms at your sides with your hands several inches apart from your hips. Relax your shoulders. Sink into your breath, as you relax and sink into the ground beneath you. Stay here for at least ten minutes—and for as long as you like beyond that. The sweet sensation that comes with this pose—with practice and with letting go—is said to be a taste of pure consciousness, of *Samadhi*-like bliss.

During this time, I also started getting more of my writing published and began teaching creative writing classes. Eventually, Neil and I were offered jobs at the University of British Columbia in Vancouver, Canada. We bought an old house that we're fixing up room by room. Lucien and Salem play together in the backyard.

Yoga and healthy eating continue to be essential for me. They are my antidepressants, my therapy, the fuel that keeps me energized and feeling good. I'd no sooner wake up on a Monday morning and have a bagel with cream cheese or a chocolate donut than knock back a beer. I practice yoga—at home, as much as I can with a young child—doing restorative poses and headstands and forward bends and meditation on some days, while on other days, a more-vigorous sequence of standing poses and backbends. I also attend an advanced Iyengar class once or twice a week.

Surrender to God brings perfection in Samadhi.

—B. K. S. Iyengar

These days I find that I don't stress out about weight and my diet like I used to; it's stopped being such a struggle. I stay mindful of how my clothes fit and make minor adjustments to my diet and exercise routine if they start getting tight, but I don't get on the scale very often. I don't waste time, like I did for so many years, wondering how my life would be better if only I could lose those extra pounds. At long last, I'm comfortable in my own skin.

I don't feel deprived, either. Over the years, my appetite and metabolism and tastes have adjusted to a yogic way of eating. I crave healthy foods and find myself jonesing for junk food and refined carbohydrates only when I'm tired or grouchy. When the craving strikes, I know that what I really need is rest—whether a restorative yoga pose, an earlier bedtime, a bath, a walk, or some guilty-pleasure television time on the couch with Salem.

I enjoy what I eat and indulge in special treats when I really want—and can appreciate—them. Rather than chowing down on a bag of chips while checking my e-mail, I'll have a small but perfect ice cream cone while sitting outside on a summer afternoon or I'll enjoy a chocolate croissant from my favorite pastry shop on a snowy day with a friend. I'm also happy to have the occasional day of very light eating. Ram Dass says that eventually the yogi will be able to live on fruit and nuts alone. I definitely don't go that far, but I can certainly see how a lighter diet can support a contemplative or spiritual life. On Saturdays, for example, when I attend my two-hour advanced yoga class, I usually skip lunch and have a big fruit breakfast in the late morning instead.

In addition to eating moderately, I try to eat as locally and seasonally as I can manage. In the spring and summer and early fall months, I do my grocery shopping at the neighborhood farmers' market near our house in Vancouver, a health-oriented city filled with hiking trails—part of the reason we decided to come here. Last summer we vacationed at a Slow Food farm on nearby Vancouver Island and ate kale from the garden with our fresh-from-the-hen-house eggs and handmade pasta. And, yes, I ate every bite! In fact, we had locally made cheese on fresh-baked baguettes for lunch everyday, and somehow I didn't gain a pound. (Must be the British Columbia paradox—spend your vacation hiking and being in nature and you can eat a cheese sandwich a day.) We'll return this summer for a week, and we're already daydreaming about the Sunday six-course vegetarian tasting lunch on the porch. (What makes this different from my old, over-the-top meals of the past is that I'll budget for it calorie-wise, eat a little less, and exercise a little more, before and after.)

Am I super-skinny? That's not my goal. I'm at a healthy and sustainable weight for me—a size 4, depending on the brand. (Side note: some brands seem to be making their clothes bigger and bigger to match the new, larger American figure. While I'm usually a 4, these days at certain stores I'm suddenly a size 2 or 0. This probably helps sell clothes, but it won't do anything to encourage health consciousness.) More important, when I happen to have a bad day (or week), I don't sink down into emotional quicksand and become depressed like I used to. The same principles of yoga philosophy that have helped me get healthy on the outside have helped me become healthy on the inside, too.

Sounds pretty good, right? Maybe, you're thinking, too good to be true?

Ever since changing my life that year in the Berkshires seven years ago, I admit to waking up some mornings and thinking, "How great is *this*." When you grow up living in fear of the next physical or verbal attack like I did, it's amazing just to feel safe and emotionally secure. To feel healthy, happy, loved, and creatively fulfilled on top of that is a blessing.

Life isn't perfect, though. Some days I do get sad thinking about my childhood, feeling the lack of grandparents in Lucien's life, and then there's the usual stress of balancing work and family. I definitely haven't morphed into some kind of a yoga saint. I do have the occasional moment of bliss—or what yogis call *samadhi*—but I also have plenty of moments of what we Long Islanders call bitchiness, too. Just ask Neil.

And, although I wish it weren't so, I know that in the future I'll face challenges more complicated and heartbreaking than learning how to lose weight and be healthy. To stay on my yogic path, I'll need to remain flexible, adjust to new circumstances, take deep breaths when I'm angry or anxious, and hug my loved ones close and tight when I'm sad. I'll have to look for moments of sun and treasure them. In between, I'll need plenty of pineapple bowls, lots of walks with Salem, and to keep my yoga mat rolled out beside me. I know that if *I* can do it—if I can go from being depressed, overweight, and borderline suicidal to just a little bit enlightened—then *you* can do it, too. Are you ready to join me?

an enLIGHTened
reading list

Mark Bittman, *How to Cook Everything Vegetarian* (Hoboken, New Jersey: John Wiley & Sons, 2007).

--------. *Food Matters: A Guide to Conscious Eating* (New York: Simon & Schuster, 2009).

Bobby Clennell, *The Woman's Yoga Book: Asana and Pranayama for All Phases of the Menstrual Cycle* (Berkeley, California: Rodmell Press, 2007).

--------. *Be Here Now* (San Anselmo, California: Hanuman Foundation, 1978).

Ram Dass, *Miracle of Love: Stories about Neem Karoli Baba* (Santa Fe, New Mexico: Hanuman Foundation, [1979] 1985).

T. K. V. Desikachar, *The Heart of Yoga: Developing a Personal Practice* (Rochester, Vermont: Inner Traditions International, 1995).

B. K. S. Iyengar, *Light on Yoga* (New York: Schocken Books, 1979).

--------. *Light on the Yoga Sutras of Patañjali* (London, England: Thorsons, 2002).

--------. *Light on Life: The Yoga Journey to Wholeness, Inner Peace, and Ultimate Freedom.* (New York: Rodale, 2005).

Geeta Iyengar, *Yoga: A Gem for Womem* (Spokane, Washington: Timeless Books, 1990).

Barbara Kingsolver, *Animal, Vegetable, Miracle: A Year of Food Life* (New York: HarperCollins, 2007).

Judith Lasater, *Relax and Renew: Restful Yoga for Stressful Times* (Berkeley, California: Rodmell Press, 2005).

Leslie McEachern, *The Angelica Home Kitchen: Recipes and Rabble Rousings from an Organic Vegan Restaurant* (New York: Round-table, 2000).

The Moosewood Collective, *Moosewood Restaurant Low-Fat Favorites* (New York: Clarkson N. Potter, 1996).

Marion Nestle, *What to Eat* (New York: North Point Press, 2006).

Michael Pollan, *In Defense of Food: An Eater's Manifesto* (New York: The Penguin Press, 2008).

Swami Prabhavananda and Christopher Isherwood, *How to Know God: The Yoga Aphorisms of Patanjali* (Hollywood, California: Vedanta Society, 2007).

Sri Swami Satchidananda, *The Yoga Sutras of Patanjali* (Yogaville, Virginia: Integral Yoga Publications, 1978).

Alisa Smith and J.B. MacKinnon, *The 100-Mile Diet: A Year of Local Eating* (Toronto, Canada: Random House Canada, 2007).

Robert Svoboda, *Ayurveda for Women: A Guide to Vitality and Health* (Rochester, Vermont: Healing Arts Press, 2000).

Linda Sparrowe with Patricia Walden, *The Woman's Book of Yoga and Health: A Lifelong Guide to Wellness* (Boston, Massachusetts: Shambhala, 2002).

Andrew Weil, *Eating Well for Optimum Health: The Essential Guide to Bringing Health and Pleasure Back to Eating* (New York: Quill, 2001).

an enLIGHTened resource list

Here's how you can find some of the yoga teachers and yoga centers mentioned in this book:

Take a class with Bobby Clennell (or with one of her fellow teachers) at the Iyengar Yoga Institute of New York, www.iyengarnyc .org/space.html, or check out Bobby's website for more on her book, her drawings, and her teaching schedule: www.bobbyclennell.com.

Patricia Walden, one of the foremost yoga teachers in North America, teaches workshops around the country, and a regular schedule of classes in Cambridge, Massachusetts. Find out more: www.yoga .com/www/patriciawalden.

My favorite teacher in L.A. is Marla Apt, who teaches at Yoga Works in Santa Monica, and at the Iyengar Yoga Institute of Los Angeles. Find out more about Marla and Iyengar yoga at www .iyila.org. Also check out Marla's class and workshop schedule: www.yoganga.com/marla.

For more information on the Jivamukti Yoga School, see www.jivamuktiyoga.com. The main center is in downtown

Manhattan—and my beloved teacher Ruth Lauer-Manenti still teaches class there—but Jivamukti-trained teachers can be found throughout North America and in Europe.

Visit the Iyengar Yoga Institute of San Francisco for yoga classes in the San Francisco Bay Area. www.iyisf.org

For more on Baron Baptiste's centers and workshops, see www.baronbaptiste.com.

Learn more about the Kripalu Center for Yoga and Health, located in Stockbridge, Massachusetts, at www.kripalu.org.

Omega Institute's main campus is in Rhinebeck, New York. For yoga and personal growth related workshops and retreats, see www.eomega.org.

Spirit Rock Meditation Center in Marin County, California offers classes, daylong programs, and residential retreats in the Vipassana Meditation tradition. See www.spiritrock.org for more information.

an enLIGHTened playlist

Check out some of my favorite musicians bringing a Western influence to spiritual yogic chanting. Download their music and experience a live *kirtan* chanting session when they tour in your city.

Krishna Das
www.krishnadas.com

Wah
www.wahmusic.com

Jai Uttal
www.jaiuttal.com

an enLIGHTened restaurant guide

Here are some of my favorite vegetarian or vegetarian-friendly restaurants around the U.S. and in my new hometown of Vancouver, Canada, where you can be sure to get a healthy and enlightened meal.

New York

Angelica Kitchen
You can't go wrong with the daily dragon bowl of lentils, veggies, and rice.

300 East 12th Street
New York, NY
(212) 228 - 2909
angelicakitchen.com

Souen
Organic and macrobiotic food

210 Sixth Avenue at Prince Street
New York, NY
(212) 807-7421

28 East 13th Street
between University Place and 5th Avenue
(212) 627-7150
souen.net

Candle Café
Vegetarian and vegan fare

1307 Third Avenue at 75th Street
New York, NY
(212) 472-0970
www.candlecafe.com

Massachusetts

Bizen Gourmet Japanese Cuisine
Beautifully and healthfully prepared Japanese food

17 Railroad Street
Great Barrington, MA
(413) 528-4343

Colorado

WaterCourse Foods
The best veggie burgers

837 E. 17th Avenue
Denver, CO 80203
(303) 832-7313
watercoursefoods.com

Los Angeles

Real Food Daily
Organic vegan cuisine (celebrity sightings, too)

514 Santa Monica Blvd.
Santa Monica, CA
(310) 451–7544

414 N. La Cienega Blvd.
Los Angeles, CA
(310) 289-9910
realfood.com

Vancouver, BC

Chutney Villa
Don't miss the South Indian vegan "Village Feast."

147 Broadway East
Vancouver, British Columbia
(604) 872-2228
chutneyvilla.com

an enLIGHTened author

JESSICA BERGER GROSS is a longtime yoga devotee and editor of the award-winning anthology *About What Was Lost: 20 Writers on Miscarriage, Healing, and Hope*. Originally from Long Island, New York, Jessica lives in Vancouver, British Columbia with her husband, their son, and Salem, their dog. She teaches creative writing at the University of British Columbia.

acknowledgments

My heartfelt thanks to my agent, Douglas Stewart, for believing in me and my writing ever since I sent him that first stack of pages years ago. Thanks, too, to Seth Fishman, also at Sterling Lord Literistic, for all his help and support. Ann Treistman, my editor at Skyhorse, was wonderful to work with; our conversations challenged me, inspired me, and made this a better book.

I wouldn't have been able to transform my life, much less write a book about it, without the guidance and inspiration of my teachers inside and outside of the yoga world. The late Sylvia Avner encouraged my love of reading. Larry Waxman, my drama teacher at South Side High School, helped me to imagine the possibility of a creative life. Thank you to Ann Klotz and her colleagues at the Ensemble Theatre Community School, including Tara Munjee, for introducing me to yoga and the power of stillness. My understanding of yoga and what it means to live a yogic life was formed by my studies at the Jivamukti Yoga Center. Thank you to Sharon Gannon and David Life for their work there and particularly to my favorite Jivamukti teacher, Ruth Lauer-Manenti, whose spiritual teachings made a huge difference at a crucial time. I am indescribably grateful for the teachings of B. K. S. Iyengar and Geeta

Iyengar and to the Iyengar method teachers with whom I've had the privilege of studying. Especially important to me has been Patrica Walden in Cambridge, Massachusetts, whose before class talks on the Yoga Sutras made them seem much less esoteric and who helped me develop my asana practice. During my pregnancy, Bobby Clennell at the Iyengar Institute in New York kept me comfortable and helped me go upside down until the very end. I am forever indebted to Bobby for contributing her beautiful illustrations to this book and for making sure my descriptions of the yoga poses are consistent with the Iyengar method. Louie Ettling in Vancouver helped me find my practice again after the birth of my son. Ellen Taylor and Linda Luz-Alterman provided wisdom, guidance, and the tools I needed to make a change.

Danielle Friedman told me I should write this book. Daphne Kalotay gave me great comments on the manuscript. Ezekiel Peterson suggested the phrase "peace, love, and pineapples." His mother, Susanna Sonnenberg, has given me advice when I needed it and helped me become a better writer. My fabulous friend Emily Barman reminded me to be kind to myself, both in recounting my experiences and in daily life. When I became overwhelmed with juggling a baby and a book deadline, Kristen Lewis urged me to keep writing; I'm so lucky to have found a friend walking the same path. Katherine Brennan has been there for me from mozzarella sticks to vegetarian chili. Her advice on teaching Lucien to nap at home made writing this book possible. Alexa Woods provided several essential hours of loving childcare each week.

For letting me share their stories and recipes I'd also like to thank my friends Jackie Kersh, Jenna Korff and her mother, Louise Marshall, Chindi Varadarajulu, and Mitchell Stevens. Many thanks to Marion Nestle for explaining to me why pineapple and *dahl baht* can help you lose weight.

It's hard to imagine this book coming to be without the love, encouragement, and day in day out support of my husband, Neil Gross. Although he'd never be caught engaging in New Age talk, the fact of the matter is that we have gone through this spiritual transformation together. He's held my hand through the hardest moments in my life and the most magical ones. Not only has Neil helped make it possible for me to write over the last several years, he has been involved in almost every aspect of this book, from brainstorming with me about the overall conception and structure to offering his ridiculously good line edits—not to mention testing out recipes, preparing healthy dinners, and taking time away from his own work to provide lots of extra childcare so that I could finish on time. Thank you, sweetie.

Love and kisses to my favorite little pineapple, Lucien. You are, of course, the best thing that's ever happened to me.

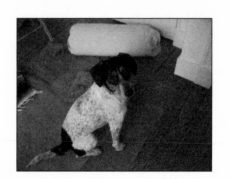